"An Emotional Abortion, or Emotionally Aborted?"

i.e.: Abortion:

A Failure to develop to completion or maturity

The premature ending or abandonment of an undertaking.

Judith Birdsong

"An Emotional Abortion, or Emotionally Aborted"
By Judith Birdsong

ISBN-13:
978-0692435946 (Judith Birdsong)
ISBN-10:
0692435948
First Edition

Cover design by Judith Birdsong

In Loving Memory
Jeremy Michael Birdsong (1973-1973)

In John 3:3, Jesus said, *"Most assuredly, I say to you, unless one is born again, he cannot see the kingdom of God."* I realize of course that this is conditional to one being born and given the opportunity to be born again, or to be born a second time. We see in Hebrews 9:27, *"And as it is appointed for men to die once, but after this the judgment."* It is clear, while we are appointed to die only once, we understand that we are to be born, or birthed twice. I realize and confess, I have mercilessly murdered my own son, Jeremy Michael Birdsong by means of abortion. I thank God and Jeremy, for their forgiveness in this unconscionable act against them both.

In John 3:5, Jesus responded to Nicodemus' question, "How can we be born a second time?" ... *"He answered, most assuredly, I say to you, unless one is born of water and the Spirit, he cannot enter the kingdom of God."* An awareness that I never allowed Jeremy to be born of the water, or the opportunity to be born a second time, will forever haunt me with relentless questions; questions that I don't know will ever be answered, at least, not until I stand before God.

In John 3:6, Jesus said, *"That which is born of the flesh is flesh, and that which is born of the Spirit is Spirit."* In this passage it is clearly defined that we are comprised of two very important components; our body, which is referred to as the flesh, and our spirit. Through this passage I see that we are conceived or created first in the womb of our mother, who carries us for 37-40 weeks. We are established by God in the womb which becomes the first training ground where we will develop, learn, grow, and thrive in our diminutive life of flesh. It is there in the womb that we learn how to eat, study, mature and exercise our muscles of flesh in preparation of the battle of our first birth and life into this fleshly realm in which we all dwell for what is recognized as just a short, whispered, fading moment in time.

Once we are born of water and come forth into the world, we continue to live in a different kind of womb. The spiritual womb! Life is yet another womb that we will spend our next several years in. In this spiritual womb, once again, we will learn how to feed ourselves, but this time our food will be spiritual food, the WORD OF GOD! With this spiritual food we will begin to thrive, grow, exercise our spiritual muscles, and be born a second time of the Spirit. Through the Spirit we will discover and prepare ourselves for a new battle, or training ground, a Spiritual battle for eternal life. Spiritual Warfare, if you will! While we operate in this training ground of life for about 70 years, give or take, we store up our heavenly rewards, the jewels of our heavenly crown, or not, the choice and free will is ours.

I know, Jeremy that I stole from you, so many opportunities in life. You will never know the experience of watching a cocoon become a butterfly, of a rose bud.....flowering, counting the stars in heaven, your first kiss, your first love, your graduation, or your wedding. You will never know fatherhood, parenting, or the nurturing love of a fleshly mother. The beauty of our fleshly experiences has been lost to you, but your gain has been so great in your experiences with our Father. I wonder Father God, did I steal from Jeremy his opportunity to be born a second time? Did I steal his opportunity to be born into the spiritual realm, while in his fleshly training ground to earn his rewards in heaven? I want to confess my awareness of just how much more I have stolen from my son, not just his life, but his opportunity to serve You, Father God. I know that he rests in the protection of Your arms, and the bosom of Your love now..... And yet, I wonder just how much I have cheated Jeremy out of, by stealing his life from him. Father, I want to offer to Jeremy the jewels of my crown that I have earned throughout my life, here in the flesh. I ask for the opportunity to earn more jewels for my crown that I may offer Jeremy even more. I know the jewels cannot make up for robbing Jeremy of his training and his life, but I want him to know that I love him enough to give up my own jewels and all that I have for him, as I would for any of my children.

Although, it seems so little to offer in return for my wrongs done to Jeremy, I know in my heart of hearts that except for my love, it is the only gift I have to offer him now, since I have stolen the gift of life from him. I offer Jeremy all the love my heart can hold and not just what my heart can hold, but with all the overflow of the love of my heart as well. I know Jeremy that you were meant to be my first born son and I have also robbed you of your inheritance therein. You were meant to be the son, born of my flesh and God's Spirit, a son that was meant to be full of life, of love, kindness, patience, joy, of great and many talents, and loyal to the service of our God. I wonder Jeremy, is there unfinished business here in the earth because I stopped you from living the life and the destiny that Almighty God Himself designed for you?

Jeremy, a day will come when I will be able to hear the joy of your laughter, the sound of your voice calling me mommy as you cry out. "I forgive you mommy," and "I love you mommy!" I long for the day, the moment when I can hold you in my arms and feel your heart beat against me once more as I squeeze you ever so gently in my arms and whisper in your ear how much I love you, my son. Together we will sing and dance with the flowers of heaven and worship our God, embracing one another! Until then Jeremy…..

All my love,
Mommy

TABLE OF CONTENTS

Acknowledgments

First and foremost, I would like to give all gratitude, glory, and praise to my Lord and Savior, Jesus Christ, the Son of my Living God! He has given me the courage, and strength to write these pages. I am eternally grateful for His direction that has led me in sound wisdom, to do His will, while planting the seeds of His mercy, His grace and His love.

I am thankful from the depth of my heart to my children, Jimmy, Jeffrey and Jeni-lee, who have not always understood the *"Why's, or What* for's" of our lives. Nonetheless, they have traveled the arid, desolate, lonely road with me which took us through many hills, valleys and mountains. They could not have realized the depth or magnitude of the underlying faults, or the lack of education that lay within the heart and soul of their mother and yet, they loved me despite my lack of knowledge, or understanding.

For my beautiful daughter, Jeni-lee, whom I have loved with my whole heart, not from the time she was conceived, mistakenly, but from the time she was born. Her struggle for emotional survival has been an amazing, miraculous feat in the world that she was born to. Her wonderful beauty, her kindness, her love for others, and her sense of compassion and forgiveness has sustained my heart through these many years. It is my prayer that the words held within the walls of these few pages will further Jeni-lee's healing, growth and understanding of the many great trials and circumstances that befell her in the beginning, not when she was born, but upon the moment she was conceived. May the grace and mercy of our Lord Jesus Christ bring her into a closer relationship, walk, and understanding of His perfect will and purpose for her life.

A special thanks for a very special woman, Debbie Granath, who has been a friend who is greater than a sister. Her emotional support, loyalty and companionship has carried me through many trials in past years.

Last but not least, I would like to thank the women of the High Desert Pregnancy Clinic in Yucca Valley, California. A special thanks to Laura Jensen and Glenda Machado, and the entire team who have offered their support, knowledge, expertise, uplifting prayers, and encouragement for success in the writing of these pages.

INTRODUCTION

Abortion was legalized in 1973. It was then, I found myself pregnant and alone, at 16 years of age. Not knowing what to do, and with great trepidation, I told my mother I was pregnant. She was very angry to say the least, and insisted I have an abortion. I was told by my mother that if I had the baby, she would disown me, leaving me to move onto the streets to have my baby there and fend for myself. She said I was an embarrassment to her and made me promise to never tell anyone, or speak of this pregnancy again.

Out of ignorance and fear, I chose to have an abortion. I never thought about it and blindly did as I was told. Five days after my abortion, I realized for the first time that I had just killed an innocent baby, and not just any baby, but my own baby. I knew at that moment I was going to hell, and nothing else mattered anymore. My heart was broken, no, it was shattered ….. shattered into tiny, irreparable fragments. A tear rolled down my cheek, and I knew I had brought this unfathomable evil upon myself. I had no right to cry anymore and so, I let the memory go, refusing to give in to the battle of acceptance. The problem was, at the time, I didn't realize just how broken my heart really was. I cried for a few minutes, sucked it up, and went on with my life for the next 40 years.

A year and a half later, I had my first child, married, divorced, remarried, and had two more children. My life became so busy, I didn't have time to mourn, or become distressed over my abortion, and so it all became a distant memory, stored in a neatly packed little parcel that I had packed away and forgot about for forty years.

Studies have revealed a little know, yet fascinating fact. From the moment of conception, the mother will carry her child's stems cells, or DNA in her body, for the rest of her life, whether her pregnancy ends in birth, miscarriage, still born, or abortion. In Genesis 4:10 God said,

An Emotional Abortion, or Emotionally Aborted?

"What have you done? The voice of your brother's blood cries out to Me from the ground."

The Hebrew word for "Blood" is "Dam" (dawm), and means guiltiness + innocent. It also means to be stopped, cut down and silenced. Is it coincidence that we call abortion, *"The Silent Holocaust?"*

DNA is found in the white blood cells, and white blood cells are found in our stem cells. Is it possible, the voice of the blood of every aborted child cries out to God, refusing to be silenced? Is it possible, that neatly packed little parcel I stored in my subconscious, contained my aborted child's stem cells, who cried out to God inside of me for 40 years?

I believe the blood of every murdered child cries out to God in his or her innocence, through the mother's memories, which will torment her until she fully comprehends and understands the depth of her sin, bringing her to repentance before God with a broken heart. In Mark 5: 2, 3, and 5 the word tells us,

2. ... immediately there met Him out of the tombs a man with an unclean spirit. 3. Who had his dwelling among the tombs; and no one could bind him, not even the chains, 5. And always, night and day, he was in the mountains and in the tombs, crying out and cutting himself with stones.

Once again, the Greek word for "Tombs" is "Mneme" (mnay may), and means remembrance, or memory. I believe these scriptures clearly show just how tormented a post abortive woman can be, whether she fully realizes it, or not. The grief and torment, although it is often self-inflicted, is enough to cause one to cut, slice, and dice their own fleshly bodies as well as their spiritual bodies. Take a moment to consider the amount of emotional pain she must be in. In fact, many post abortive women are cutters, alcoholics, drug addicts, not to mention a great many post abortive women suffer from various mental illnesses, including depression and P.A.S.

Not only are more than a million babies a year being murdered, but equally as many, or more, men and women are murdered emotionally and spiritually because of their sin of abortion and unforgiveness of themselves. If they can't forgive themselves, then how can they ever believe God will forgive them? Most post abortive men and women are consumed with guilt, shame, grief, anger, pain, confusion, uncertainty, and fear as they walk the earth in a fog, or the disillusionment of life. These men and women need your love first, and then your understanding. To do this successfully, you need to know and understand the emotional pain that inhabits her heart, brought on by the crying out of the blood of the innocent that remains in her body throughout her lifetime.

The symptoms of post abortive men and women infects every area of their lives, including, but not limited to:

Relationships	Friends	Love
Marriage	Acquaintances	Trust
Children	Jobs	Sleep
Siblings	Successes	
Parents	Failures	

I am sharing my story with you, in the hope of helping others to see that; there is nothing man can make, no pill, no medication, no treatment, or counselor that can heal a broken, or shattered heart. It is only the supernatural love of God that can heal the tragedy of a broken heart. There is hope for every post abortive woman and man, if you will but open the eyes of your heart, and see the light that lies ahead.

Healing and forgiveness has finally come for me as I pray it does for the millions, and millions of men and women out there, who are still walking in their broken and shattered hearts, or *"Post Abortive Syndrome,"* better known as P.A.S. Luke 4:18 tells us exactly why Jesus came,

"*He has sent Me to heal the brokenhearted, to proclaim liberty to the captive and recovery of sight to the blind, to set at liberty those who are oppressed...*"

Chapter 1

A Stolen Generation

I sat quietly upon the edge of my bed one afternoon, surrounded by the study materials and books I had been collecting for the last several years. I stared at the potpourri of posted scriptures and crosses that created a collage on the walls of the small, confining room, where I temporarily resided. Before long, I began to wander in one of the many chambers of my mind. As I jumped from chamber to chamber in the echoes of my memories, my thoughts wrestled against each other in search of an answer….. An answer that would explain why I was still living in the captivity and bondage of financial ruin.

I shivered in the brisk air as a draft brushed across my shoulder, and I looked at the small, dark window that seemed to be tucked away, hiding from the warmth of the light. It was a cold November afternoon, and a chilly wind blew over the valley. I wondered why God had not yet released me from this spiritual desert I had been living in for the last four years, when suddenly, I was stirred from my thoughts by the ringing chimes of my cell phone.

I reached for the phone and answered to hear a soft, childlike voice on the other end and to my surprise, it was my eldest granddaughter, Aryana.

With a quickened rush of excitement, I imagined her big brown eyes lighting up in my mind as she exclaimed, "Hi Grandma, it's me, Aryana." It had only been a couple of months since I taught her to memorize my phone number, in the event of an emergency.

Because it was a school day, I curiously asked, "Aryana, where are you calling me from?"

Aryana exclaimed excitedly, "I am at school with my sister, grandma." I could hear the excitement of accomplishment in her tone. This was the first time she had called since memorizing my phone number. I realized something was very wrong for her to call me from school.

I could hear my youngest granddaughter, Savannah, speaking in the background and laughing at her own nonsensical comments. Savannah was a little clown who loved to laugh and make others laugh as well. Savannah and Aryana were just under eleven months apart in age, and in many aspects they acted as twins, and yet they are as different as night and day.

The two sisters are very competitive with each other, but would defend one another with their last breath, sticking together as though they had been glued to one another. Even so, my eldest granddaughter, Aryana, is an overly compassionate, free spirited, strong willed, and very determined little girl. She carries a leading personality and always manages to see the good and endless possibilities in everything around her. My youngest granddaughter, Savannah, is a very emotionally charged, a little bit silly, and a very personable young lady with a touch of perfectionism. Little did either of them realize, they were about to be taken from their home, family, and everything that was familiar to them.

Aryana, still on the phone, continued to speak quickly and assertively, "I am at my school with the CPS lady and she wants to talk to you. Do you want to talk to her, Grandma?" Before I could respond with a yes, or a no, Aryana repeated her words with more intensity.

"She wants to talk to you, okay Grandma?"

My hand squeezed tightly around the phone as I felt my jaw bear down, clamping tightly. Attempting to speak, I said, "Okay, I love you sweetheart and don't you worry," fighting to disguise the surprise and dread that fell on my heart at that moment.

A woman's voice spoke guardedly and hesitantly, introducing herself by name as a social worker with, "Children's Protective Services," or better known as "CPS." She explained that she was at the school following up on a report made to CPS by an anonymous caller. The report stated that my granddaughters were suffering from parental neglect. I was informed that she had found sufficient reason to believe my granddaughters were being neglected.

"After watching the girls for the last few days, and speaking with both of them today, I have determined that both of the girls should be removed from their mother's home and care," she stated without emotion.

My heart began to race when I heard her ask, "Are you able to pick up your granddaughters, and keep them with you indefinitely, or until this situation can be resolved? Otherwise, I will have no choice but to take them into custody, and place them into a foster home."

I leapt to my feet in surprise as my mind launched into a psychological frenzy. My thoughts were scrambling to find a way to protect and defend, as only a mother would do. I had to think of a way to keep this from happening. Was it possible that this woman could step in and take my granddaughters from their Mother? ...From me? ...From their family? "This couldn't be happening," I thought to myself. "This isn't real!" The thought pounded against the pinnacles of my mind as my heart began to beat rapidly.

Everything felt so surreal. Any minute now, this CPS worker was going to tell me that everything was okay, and this has all been a big mistake. God wouldn't let this happen, not to me... Not to my daughter... Not to my family... and certainly not to my granddaughters! How could this be? I had spent the last four years praying for my children, and my children's, children. I stood daily for their salvation, deliverance, healing, happiness, and success in their lives.

I had especially prayed for my daughter, Jeni-lee and interceded for her sobriety. Upon every given opportunity, I had witnessed to her about our Lord Jesus, and how much He loved her. I explained to her the great miracles God could, and would do for her, if only she would just surrender her life to Him. I had even reminded her of how much she once loved Jesus as a child. Although, it seemed everything I said to her was futile, I also understood that every word was a seed planted in her body, spirit, and her soul. All she needed now was the watering for the seeds to begin to sprout and grow.

I knew God's saving grace would deliver Jeni-lee from the clutches of all that was evil. I believed He would deliver her from the generational curses, and from her inevitable death by her own hand, whether deliberate, or by unintentional suicide. I knew God would deliver her from the addictions of her drug and alcohol use, and from her life destroying anger, unforgiveness and self-mutilation. He would also deliver her from the spirit of death, rebellion, rejection, and abandonment that pressed upon Jeni-lee, not from the time of her birth, but from conception, from deep within the womb in which she grew, so many years ago.

Didn't God promise me that if I were saved, my household would also be saved? Scriptures began to flash through my mind as I recalled the words in Acts. Paul said in Acts 16:31,

"And they answered, Believe on the Lord Jesus Christ, and you will be saved, you and your household."

I stood clutching the phone to my ear as I nervously paced the floor. I vigorously walked while I desperately searched my heart for the words, and God's will to speak with the CPS worker. I asked her about the circumstances that led to this phone call. "Why? What is going on? Why are you taking my granddaughters?"

"I came to the school where your granddaughters attend, to interview both of them, individually and together. After visiting the home and speaking with your granddaughters today, I believe their mother is using drugs. Savannah tells me, she saw her mother smoking brown cigarettes, clearly stating that she knows her mother smokes marijuana. Both girls have also stated, they have seen their mother drinking alcohol, revealing to me, in their own words, 'She doesn't get drunk anymore and fall down.' They also complained that their mother sleeps all the time."

She continued, "Both girls have said, they don't get enough to eat, and sometimes there isn't a lot of food. I have visited the home and noticed there was little food in the home, but they were not without."

The very center of my being shook before God... "Please, don't let this happen. Please Father God, tell me this isn't so, please, please, please, I pleaded!"

I argued, explaining to this cautious, but sternly spoken woman that I had visited my daughter's home just a few days ago in response to a call from my daughter for help with groceries. A friend took us shopping and purchased groceries for her and the girls, totaling nearly $300. We stocked her kitchen with healthy, planned meals. I know there is food in the house and the girls were getting plenty to eat.

I stopped to draw my next breath when the CPS worker's unflinching voice broke through, stating, "Ms. Birdsong, your granddaughters, individually, have voiced to me that they both want to live with you." Again, she asked, "Will you be able to come and pick up your granddaughters from the school, and keep them with you until we can resolve these issues?"

She informed me, it was always the goal of CPS to reunite the mother with her children, whenever possible. "We have an abundance of various plans of action, and lists of counseling programs that would help Jeni-lee. We will also cover whatever expenses are incurred for medical, or treatment plans for her," she said.

A dead silence followed her impatient and final words as they resounded like an echo in the back of my mind. I resigned myself to having to explain to her some very personal details about my life.

I became fearful that she wouldn't have the patience to listen to what I had to tell her, or she would think I was making excuses. My spirit cried out to God, confused and afraid, begging Him to tell me what to do, or say, to stop all of this nonsense. I suppose, I knew all along this day was inevitable. The consistent poor choices my daughter continually made, would eventually cost us all, very dearly. I didn't want to believe, it was no longer just a fear, but a reality. I had no deck to draw my cards from and decided to shorten my story, speaking quickly. Hopefully she would be merciful, and give my daughter another chance. In the back of my mind, I cried out, *"Dear Jesus, help me,"* as I stood very still, drawing in another deep breath.

Panicking, I blurted out, "Okay, here it is! Let me make a very long story, as short as I can, if you will just give me a minute. I cannot pick my granddaughters up right now. I have nowhere to take them. I lost everything, and have absolutely nothing left. I am staying with my son and his wife, because I don't have my own home at this time.

"Please," I said, hesitating a moment. "About four years ago, I became very ill and shortly thereafter, for all intents and purposes, I should have died. I survived three days on life support, and was very ill for the next three years. Being a widow, I think it goes unsaid, I lost everything."

Attempting to capture her understanding and compassion, I continued, "By everything, I mean, I lost my job, my car, my home, my credit, and every opportunity for financial gain. As a result, I have been left without a place to live. I have been living in complete faith in God, to heal me and supply my needs. At this time in my life, I can't do anything for myself, or of myself, although, I have not given up, and I am still battling to change my circumstances."

I continued to explain, "When I came to stay with my son and daughter in law, she made it explicitly clear to me that she didn't want my granddaughters at her house, not even to visit. While I am not completely whole, my health is improving a little more each day, and I am already much better than I have been. I am still unemployed with physical limitations, and I am searching diligently for employment. In this suffering economy, I haven't had many opportunities, but I am still very hopeful. I desperately wish things were different, but I just don't have my own home, or a safe, welcoming place to take my granddaughters at this time."

Embarrassed, I asked if they had any programs to help me take the girls, and provide a safe environment for them. I was determined to not let pride stand in the way of my family, as I explained how much I wanted to take the girls into my custody, to love and care for them.

"The state will pay Foster Parents to care for my grandchildren. Would they be able to help me? Would they help to place me into a low income residence? If they could help with housing, I would be willing to apply for state aid while I set up our home, find child care and return to work as soon as possible," I said, bargaining with her and finally I pleaded, "I would be willing to do anything at all to keep my family together."

"There are no programs to help with living arrangements for you and your granddaughters," she emphatically stated. She said there was nothing that she was aware of, that would help me to get and maintain custody of my granddaughters.

For a moment I was miffed by the idea that the state could, and would, forcibly take legal custody of my granddaughters. They would give money and unlimited resources to total strangers to provide for my granddaughters, yet, they would do absolutely nothing to help, or assist a grandmother, who adored and loved them.

It just didn't make sense to me! All I asked for, was a helping hand up, and a little assistance. CPS had determined to forfeit Aryana and Savannah to outsiders, offering these complete strangers any and every available assistance and resource, with pay. This was done in Lieu of helping a grandmother provide them with the knowledge that they are deeply loved, cherished and treasured. A grandmother who desired to establish a sound, fruitful, moral, and God based relationship, filled with enough love to fill the vastness of all of space and time.

There was a moment of silence between us while she contemplated my words. Then she asked, "Do you have another phone number where I can reach Jeni-lee?"

I had completely poured my heart to this woman. She blatantly disregarded every word, and I felt like my words were a left over, to be tossed into a garbage disposal and made to disappear.

"I've been calling her and there is no answer," she continued. "I have called her from both, the school's landline and my cell phone. You would think a parent would answer the phone when they see the school is calling, while their children are in attendance," she said irritated, as her impatient arrogance settled into our conversation.

Disregarding her failure to acknowledge anything I had just said, I continued to be polite, responding to her in a positive manner.

"My daughter doesn't have a phone of her own. The number you are calling is her roommate's cell number. Therefore, answering the phone is not always an option for her. Her roommate, quite often does not answer his phone, and his voicemail is full, rendering us unable to leave a message. All anyone can do, is keep calling that number until somebody eventually answers the phone," I insisted.

"I will be taking your granddaughters into custody. Hopefully, I will have them placed into a foster home by this evening," she said. "I will try to go by Jeni-lee's home since she needs to know that I have her children in custody," she bluntly spoke, clearly vexed.

Completely frustrated, I assured her, I would keep calling until I eventually reached my daughter. My mind swirled in the "What if's." What if I couldn't reach her? What if I couldn't find her? What if something happened to her? What if she can't get the girls back? I panicked at the thought of never seeing my granddaughters again, as my thoughts surged relentlessly through my mind.

I threw my head back in an attempt to regain composure, and asked where she would be taking my granddaughters. She assured me, they would be taken somewhere local, because Jeni-lee, being the mother, still had rights.

"Jeni-lee has lots, and lots of rights," she sarcastically proclaimed aloud. "Aryana and Savannah will be held at an undisclosed location with a foster family and Jeni-lee will be provided with contact information, once they reached her by phone."

The worker briefly explained, the mother of the children would have visitation rights, and they would help her with parenting classes. "We will assess her needs, to determine what we can do to reunite the family," she said, confirming once more that reunification was their primary goal. She hurriedly informed me, she had to get back to my granddaughters.

I assured her, my line was open, and I would be available if she needed to contact me, or needed my assistance for anything at all. I heard the line disconnect and the silent emptiness consumed my heart, as I pressed "End call."

Feeling exhausted by the enormous burden that had just been placed on my shoulders, the pangs of co-dependency wrestled to overtake my thoughts and emotions. My first reactions were fear and anxiety. I had a sense of urgency to find my daughter, and tell her of this terrible event that had just occurred. I feared it would cause Jeni-lee to reach a breaking point that would bring her to her own fatal demise.

I had been taking care of my daughter and granddaughters for so long now, that I was terrified at not being able to fix the problem, and simultaneously, I was afraid of being able to fix the problem. I knew if what the worker had said was true, my daughter would have to learn to properly care for her own children, and resolve her own problems. For the first time, I realized, while Jeni-lee may be my daughter, she is no longer my little girl, or a child. I knew I had to let her go now, but how? I am her mother. How do I do this? "Dear Jesus, help me," I cried aloud!

I knew I had no control over this situation, but I needed to find Jeni-lee to tell her that her children had just been appropriated by CPS. She would have to grasp the idea that her parenting rights had just been temporarily suspended. Confused and frightened, I dialed the message number for her. How do I tell my daughter, a mother, she has lost her children? I wondered how she would react to the news. I knew it wouldn't go well, no matter how I told her.

The phone rang three or four times with each call, and every call ended with a voice recording, telling me the voice mail box I was trying to reach was full. I was unable to leave any messages for her. I could only keep trying. Every phone call ended with the same recording. I called so many times, I was sure the phone was going to explode. I stared at my surroundings, hoping someone would answer my next call. I continually prayed, asking Jesus for help, patience, and the strength to continue on in my quest to complete the task that was now at hand. "Please God, let somebody answer the phone this time," I prayerfully asked.

I called the number one more time, trusting the Lord for an answer. To my astonishment, a woman's voice, not belonging to my daughter, answered the phone with a hesitant "Hello?"

I glanced down to my cell phone to be sure I had dialed the right number and abruptly answered back.

"Hello, this is Jeni-lee's mother. Is she there, or near you by chance? Please, I really need to speak with her," I pleaded. "This is a family emergency concerning her daughters."

The young lady on the phone said that neither Jeni-lee, nor her roommate were home, explaining that this message phone had been left with her in hopes she could repair an internet issue. She asked if she could help in some way, and asked what had happened. I told her I needed to speak directly with my daughter. The pleasant individual said that Jeni-lee had gone to the welfare office to apply for benefits at the CPS worker's recommendation. She didn't know when Jeni-lee or her roommate would return.

I made the decision to relay some information to the young woman. As I spoke, she interrupted, telling me the worker had already come by, spoke with her, and left a business card on Jeni-lee's door; as notification that she had taken custody of her daughters. I left a message for Jeni-lee to call me back, before hanging up. I wanted to relay the information, detailed to me by the CPS worker that I had spoken with earlier, directly to Jeni-lee myself.

Everything I could do, had been done now. All that was left to do, was wait for a return call. Waiting anxiously, I wondered how Aryana and Savannah were reacting to this. Did they understand everything that had just happened? Were they frightened? Would this emotionally traumatize them for the rest of their lives? Do they feel loved, and do they know how much I love then? The endless questions tore at my heart, and ripped through the chambers of my mind as a tornado would tear through a neighborhood, reaping havoc and laying waste, our hopes, our dreams, and our futures. The fear of a future without my precious, beautiful granddaughters, decimated my dreams of grandeur as a grandmother.

I knew I had to place all my faith, trust and hope in the Lord God, for the welfare and protection of my children, my children's children, and myself.

Darkness fell over the room as I tried to prepare myself for Jeni-lee's reaction, when I told her Aryana and Savannah were gone. Would she be angry, or enraged? I was afraid that she somehow, would blame me for this. I wondered myself, what could I have done differently?

It was approaching dinner time, and I still had not heard from Jeni-lee. I went into the washroom and turned the water on. Leaning over the basin, I cupped my hands under the flowing water, splashing the refreshingly cool water against my face to rinse away the salty tears that stung my eyes. I reached for the soft hand towel, to pat myself dry. I returned to the sofa, poising myself in preparation of relaying the horrible news to my son. He was expected to return home from work anytime.

A sudden noise startled me from the depth of silence. In my excitable state, I leapt from my poised position on the sofa, to my feet, in one swift stroke. As I stood trembling, I realized the phone was ringing. I quickly snatched it up to look at the caller I.D. It was a restricted number. Assuming it was CPS once again, I quickly pressed the phone to my ear and answered "Hello."

Again, I heard the small child like voice calling out, "Hi grandma, it's me." Aryana's voice, broken, frustrated, and weary broke through.

I knew immediately, my precious Aryana was desperately trying to be the tower of strength for herself, and her little sister, as she so often did. I could hear in Aryana's perplexed voice, she knew she could not protect her little sister this time. I listened to Savannah, sobbing hysterically in the back ground. She was crying so hard that I could hear her trying to catch her breath behind every howl of agony that sprung forth from her small lungs. Fear filled the atmosphere, and was released anew with every sobbing howl, leaving her breathless and struggling for her next gasp of air. I could hear her disheartened shrieks of broken, almost illegible words, "MOMMY, MOMMY, MOMMMMMYYYYY!"

I fought back my own tears, listening intently to my traumatized granddaughters crying out for their mommy, or their grandma to come for them. These precious little girls did not understand why I could not come for them. They were frightened, and feeling abandoned after being taken from school, the one place where they should feel safe. They had absolutely nothing familiar to surround, or comfort themselves with. Their clothes were removed by strangers. They were bathed and put into clean clothes that did not belong to them, in a stranger's home, nearly two hours away from their own home. They were surrounded by new parents, new foster siblings, unfamiliar beds, and furnishings. There were all kinds of new strangers telling them what to do, and what not to do.

"Hi baby, are you okay? Aryana, I love you so, so much! I am so sorry this has happened to you, and your sister. Don't worry sweetheart, you will be seeing mommy and grandma very soon," I promised her. With all I could muster up, I spoke to her with a calm, comforting voice as I gently asked, "What is wrong with your sister, why is she crying like that?"

I don't know grandma. Uummm..... She wants mommy and she won't stop crying," Aryana murmured in a low, withdrawn, fuzzy voice, filled with fear and confusion. Aryana, in her brokenness, fought back her own tears. She told me nobody could make Savannah stop crying.

"I can't make her stop, grandma, she just keeps crying and screaming for mommy," Aryana said, with her small voice. Her words trailed into long, silent pauses behind each word spoken aloud. It was obvious, she was struggling to be strong for her sister and struggling with her own emotions.

"Everything is going to be okay, Aryana. Do you want me to talk to your sister? Let me talk to her, my sweet princess. I love you so, so much," I softly replied.

Another voice came on the phone. It was the CPS worker. She told me, they were not able to calm Savannah down, and asked if I would speak with her to bring solace. "Savannah has made herself ill from crying hysterically," she said. I told her I would speak with her, and asked her to put Savannah on the phone.

"Savannah, Savannah, SAVANNAH," I lovingly called out, softly elevating my voice each time, attempting to get her attention. I continued to call her name, hoping she would hear me over her gasping screeches for her mother. "What is wrong sweetheart? Why are you crying?" I asked her. "It will be okay, I promise you," I said, in an effort to calm her! I love you so much baby girl, please, don't cry, its okay now," I said, attempting a note of cheer in my tone! "Hey, listen to grandma and don't cry anymore. Do you hear me, Savannah? I promise you, everything is going to be okay. You will see mommy and grandma in just a couple of days, okay?" She continued to wail and sob relentlessly in my ear as I stood there with my eyes closed, fighting back my own tears. "Savannah, my sweet girl, remember what grandma told you? If we all pray and ask Jesus to help us, He will, because He loves us so much! Be sure you remember to pray the way grandma taught you Savannah." I whispered to Jesus in the back of my mind, *"Please, Lord Jesus, Help my granddaughter."* I opened my eyes, and spoke into the phone gently but firmer this time, "Savannah, stop crying now, it's going to be alright. Do you hear me? Okay, Savannah? I promise you will see us in just a couple of days."

Suddenly, I heard Savannah's voice break through saying, "O(gasp)kay, grand(gasp)ma," followed by a long drawn out squeal of anguish. Again, she attempted to speak. "O(gasp)kay, O(gasp)kay, I (gasp) love (gasp) you (gasp) too," she said with long, soft, deep sobs, following her silence.

The CPS worker came back on the phone. "Thank you, I think she will be alright now. I have found a place for the girls temporarily and they will both be fine here. I will get them settled in now, and again, thank you," she said, sounding frazzled to the core.

"WAIT," I called out firmly. "Please, put Aryana back on the phone for just a moment. I need to speak with her again," I broke in, before she hung up. I heard a rustling sound in the phone and then silence.

"Aryana, are you okay?" I asked.

She replied with a fragile, drawn out, "Yes, grandma, I'm okay."

I assured her of how much I love her and Savannah, promising her, it would be just a couple of days before we would see each other again. I reminded Aryana to pray with her sister and ask Jesus to help us. "I love you, Aryana."

"Okay Grandma, I have to go now. I love you, bye," and silence came over the phone. How was I ever going to tell Jeni-lee about this phone call? I couldn't! It would devastate her, as it just did me. I dreaded telling my daughter, more than ever. My tears flowed, uncontrollably. Small sobs were slipping from my throat as I fought to control them. This wasn't over yet. I still had calls to make and people to talk to. I couldn't fall apart and become incoherent now.

I returned to the washroom to splash my face with cold water, once again, to remove the salty tears from my flesh, shocking me back from this new trauma that stared me in the face.

Returning to the living room, I decided to call and see if Jeni-lee had returned home. The same female voice answered the phone. I asked politely, "I was just wondering if you have heard anything from Jeni-lee yet?"

"Yes, she is right her, hold on and I will get her." She replied.

After a moment Jeni-lee came to the phone, "Hello," her voice filled with clear anticipation.

"Jeni-lee, it's mom," I blurted out. "Have you heard from the girls?" I told her in detail, what the girls had said when they called from school, and then what the worker had said. I told her, CPS had taken Aryana and Savannah into their custody, placing them into a foster home.

"Nuh-Uh," she replied in adamant denial. "They can't do that! I was at the welfare office doing everything they told me to do. Why would they do this?" Her voice bolted. "Mom, I returned home to a card on my door and my neighbor said they took my kids!" She frantically belted out. "I did everything they asked. I was at the welfare office all day today. How could they do this to me? I applied for assistance, and was assigned a really good worker today. She gave me a card with a lot of food stamps on it, so I can get food for the girls right away. While I was out doing what they said to do, they went to the school and took my girls," she said, her voice frantic, yelling and nearing hysteria.

Jeni-lee had called the numbers on the card, and the office was closed. She couldn't reach anybody to find out about Aryana and Savannah. She was panicked, tearful and screaming one minute, and fighting to regain composure the next. Despite her battle to not cry, her tears flowed endlessly.

"The CPS office recording says they are only open Monday through Thursday, four days a week, with three day weekends and no way to reach them. It is Thursday now and I can't reach them. Oh my God! Where are my daughters, they must be completely freaked out. I know Savannah is screaming for me, mom, Oh My God! What am I going to do?" She screamed hysterically into the phone.

With trembling hands and a broken voice, I tried to calm her. I didn't dare tell her about my conversation with the girls, earlier today.

Jeni-lee screamed, "If they take my daughters, I am going to kill myself! I don't have anything to live for," she cried!

She was distraught, and I didn't know how to comfort her. I reassured her, this was temporary, and everything would be alright. I had to do or say something to calm her. I was petrified at the thought of losing my daughter, and both of my granddaughters. I begged her not to hurt herself. I tried to encourage her, by telling her that she was all her daughter's had to live for. I reminded her that I had spoken with both of the girls in the past half hour. I felt I had to lie, telling her both the girls wanted their mommy, but were handling everything well, and would be just fine. With that being said, Jeni-lee calmed down enough for me to talk to her again.

"Wait," I exclaimed. I have a number the CPS worker left with me. She said if it were an emergency, we could call, and they would not give out the worker's cell number, but would put our call through to them. I think this is considered an emergency. I attempted to keep her calm, all the while, desperate to keep myself on an even keel without breaking into tears myself. With words of encouragement and promises that everything would work out, I tried to break through her renewed hysteria. I shouted over her frenzied voice as I read off the CPS worker's phone number. I wasn't sure she was hearing anything I was saying. I repeatedly asked her if she heard me, until I got a response.

Jeni-lee sharply repeated the area code and phone number back to me, saying she would call me back as soon as she knew anything. Without hesitation, not wanting to lose precious moments in finding her daughters, she hung up the phone.

I walked to the living room window, staring out to the street, as I prayed God would intervene with a great miracle, turning this around, for the sake of all of us.

My phone rang and it was Jeni-lee again. Her teeth were frantically set on edge as she screamed, "They can't do this! Where are my daughters? Oh my God, I just know Savannah is screaming for me, and Aryana, what about Aryana, mom? What am I going to do? I can't reach anyone until Monday when the office re-opens."

I didn't have any answers for her, or even for myself. I could not believe they could come and take your children from school, and because they could not reach you, leave a business card on your door, notifying you they have taken your children, and then disappear for days. It didn't seem humane! I could only imagine the turmoil in my daughter's heart. Suddenly, silence filled my ears and she calmly said, "Oh well, I have to go now, mom!" With those words she hung up the phone and it was silent once more.

I was frightened and alone. My heart was shattered and I knew without a doubt, I was absolutely helpless. There was nothing I could do to fix this, and yet, I had to remain strong for my family. I sunk into the sofa, as the warm, tingling, salty tears stung my flesh, continuously streaming over my cheeks, and falling into my lap. How could this have happened? Was this my doing? Was I really such a bad mother?

My son Jeffrey, and his wife returned home from work, driving up at the same time. I could not bring myself to talk about this ongoing dilemma. I just didn't see how talking about it was going to help my granddaughters, my daughter, or myself. I told Jeffrey that CPS had taken his nieces away from his sister. He looked at me searchingly, and dropped his gaze downward while he sat in silence, feeling helpless.

"Well, I'm not surprised," my daughter in law venomously spewed.

Agitated and not understanding her lack of compassion toward Jeni-lee, or myself, I retreated to my room and sat alone in the quiet.

I recalled the years past, recounting my hard labor, long hours, and desperate attempts to support my children, offering them what little opportunities in life, I could. I was a single, low income mom. I knew I was not a perfect mom and had made many bad choices, but I also knew I had tried harder than so many other mother's, to be as perfect as I could be. I was sure, if I stayed positive, and if I tried hard enough, it would result in perfect children, a perfect family unit and a perfect life. After all, I was a perfectionist and if I did everything as perfectly as possible, I would be strongly envied, for having the perfect relationship with my children, and the perfect family. I had known for some years now, my children, myself, and our lives were as far from perfect as the west is from the east. I suppose, I didn't realize, just how imperfect things had become. Suddenly, it seemed as though I had destroyed everything, including our future as a family. I didn't know how, but I did know that this somehow fell upon my shoulders, since my children's dad, had been out of their lives from early childhood. After all, my daughter wouldn't be an uneducated, high school dropout, or an angry addict, if only I had been a better mother. If only I had trained her up better, or, or, or..... The if's, and the or's, endlessly continued to flow in my mind as I began blaming myself for everyone's failures.

My mind continued to wonder through the foggy valley of the, what if's, of life. What if I had worked less, spent more time with her, and loved her more? What if I hadn't been so strict? What if this, and what if that? Searching for a diversion from these self-condemning, life sentencing, without parole, thoughts that ripped through my heart. My eyes turned toward the small table in front of me. I stood there staring at a poem I had written a couple of years earlier that lay across the top of the table. I began to whisper the poem aloud.....

"Tears of Sorrow"

I have wept many tears of unfulfilled sorrow,
Hoping still that my deliverance will be on the morrow...

I have laid upon mine face and called to thee with all my might,
And it was there that I watched as my soul set into flight.....

Perhaps I have not knelt in reverence as I know I should,
Since my Redeemer hung for me on that piece of wood.....

Please do not leave or forsake me in my gray headed time of need,
For I know that it is this for which my Savior was sent to bleed.....

I cried out to my Savior with this tear stained face,
As my body swayed to and fro reveling in the dance of all His grace.....

For it is through His love, His blood, and His tears,

That I may know through Him, freedom without tears
or fears…..

Suddenly, a wave of fear and emptiness washed over me, as I realized my failure as a mother. I was swirling in a vortex of emotions as the prolonged, reverberating, twisted echoes of my daughter, and my granddaughter's cries filled my heart. My own helpless torment was swallowing me alive. The reality of the depth of this overwhelming, emotional pain, struck me like a rod across my heart, knocking me to the floor and on my knees. I bowed down before my God, praying, calling out to Jesus, "Please Jesus, help me to save my children," as I continued to kneel in my brokenness, drowning in my own tears, and suffocating in every fear, laid open across my heart. I didn't want to be afraid anymore, "Please God, help me to not be afraid anymore," I sobbed with my face twisted in torment and grief.

I wept so hard, my flesh closed in tightly, banding itself across my forehead. It felt as though my head were in a vice, clamped tightly against my skull, grinding against me. I squeezed my hands over my head in an attempt to relieve the pain, as I struggled to catch my next breath. I cried out with a fragmented heart, "Why, God? Why? I don't understand, why this is happening? Was I really such a bad mother?"

"I loved my children, and I tried to be a good mother," I cried out, attempting to justify myself before God. I declared aloud, "I worked hard, I fought hard, and I loved hard for them. What did I do wrong? Please tell me what I did wrong," I pleaded! "Show me what to do now, what am I going to do now, Lord?"

I struggled to steady my breathing as I wiped my eyes, and picked myself up from the floor. Slowly, while meditating in the surreal shadows of time, I moved to sit on the edge of my bed. I remained there in prayer, while drowning in the tears that still leaked not only from my eyes, but from my heart also.

It was then, I heard His voice, so very clearly, as He said to me.....

"God is not a man that He should lie, nor a son of man that He should repent. Has He said, and He will not do? Or has He spoken, and will He not make it good?

Without interruption, He continued,

"Judith, my daughter, I have heard your cries, and I have loved you so very much. I have spent these years calling for you to return to Me."

He spoke again saying,

"You chose to spend these years in rebellion against Me. Do you remember so many years ago, when you became angry with Me, When you unrighteously judged Me, ... Me, your God? You turned your back on Me and walked away, blaming Me for your various trials and losses, brought upon you by your own lack of knowledge, your rebellion, and your sins! When you did this, My daughter, you took your children with you. You removed them out from under the umbrella of My protection, along with yourself,"

He whispered to me with such a depth of love.

"Because you have asked Me, I am faithful to forgive. Because you have invited Me, I am faithful to return. Because you have inquired of Me, I am faithful to answer, and because you have petitioned Me, I am faithful to save."

God continued to confirm to me.

"Follow Me, and I will show you how you have opened the doors for evil to overtake you, and your children, that you may understand. Follow me now that I may teach you how to close these doors. You will learn and understand my precepts. Come with Me now, my daughter, to the beginning. Let Me show you what you did wrong. Do you remember these great many years ago, when you kneeled beside your bed in prayer, and you held a knife to your heart…..

Chapter 2
An Emotional Abortion

I stood in the living room of our small two bedroom mobile home, listening to the wind howl through the window, as I gazed out into the desert with its picturesque views. Large fluffy clouds plumed over the desert scene, ornamenting the heavens with streams of sunlight, piercing through the small breaks in the obscured skies. Thunder bellowed across the thick dampness of the cactus laden sand, landscaping the desert horizon. The smell of wet sand mingled with the aroma of chicken frying on the stove top, as I prepared dinner.

Christmas was nearing, and a consuming loneliness was settling its raunchy haunches across my already heavily burdened shoulders, as a weighty depression settled on my heart. I listened to Jimmy, who is my spry, mischievous, six year old son, making race car sounds, while playing quietly in his room with his little brother. I peeked in to check on them as dinner simmered. Jeffrey was my shy, contented two year old, who's dimpled, coyish smile grabbed the ladies hearts. They had amongst them an adequate selection of toys and various learning tools to keep them busy while I made dinner.

My thoughts drifted off toward Michael, and the repressed emotions of repeated abandonment from the man I loved so much. My love for him consumed me, while my thoughts left me wondering when he would return home again. I had been living with Michael, the love of my life, and the father of our son Jeffrey, and step father to Jimmy for six years now. Michael was a tall dark, muscular framed man, whom the ladies found especially sexy and attractive. He was exceedingly intelligent and well educated, coming from a fairly affluent background. He had a sensuous wit along with a rich sense of humor, and yet, there always seemed to be a mystery about him. Michael was well liked and people in general, were drawn to him because of his intimate smile and generous heart.

It seemed, all our troubles were centered on his two mistresses, alcohol and drugs. Michael was an agnostic binge drinker, and I was a Jesus loving, codependent caretaker. Whenever Michael disappeared on one of his benders, he would slip out in the night as we all slept, never taking with him a change of clothes, or even a toothbrush. This was his way of telling me, he would be returning when he was finished partying. He would usually be gone anywhere from three days to three months. His time was usually spent with other women who would help him to consume more alcohol and, or drugs. We were closing in on the holiday season and were hopeful he would come home for Christmas.

When Michael quietly took leave of us and our home, he would take with him our only transportation. He would gather to himself all of our monthly savings, including rent and grocery money, to finance his party adventures. The children and I were left behind, abandoned and alone, to fend for ourselves. The closest store was a small country market, five miles away. It would be a ten mile trek on foot to purchase a gallon of milk. Bewildered, as to why he would do this, we would be left to wonder if he really loved us at all. On this particular occasion, Michael had been gone for nearly three months, and the children and I were beginning to miss him terribly.

Despite his shortcomings, I loved Michael from the very bowels of my heart. I didn't think it possible for any woman to love any man, more than I loved him. I believed him to be my soul mate, and I was sure I would not continue to breathe without him. I had no reason to live without him. Besides, I thought to myself, "I will never lose him, because when he's done drinking, he always comes home to me."

I came to believe, if given enough time, I could fix our lives and make him stop drinking. Whatever our problems were, I knew that if I asked Jesus to help us, and to save him, he would be faithful to hear my pleas. The problem was, I had been asking Jesus to save Michael for six years.

I believed I was strong enough to carry the burdens alone. At times, it seemed so overwhelmingly difficult, to stand all alone in the relentless drama that constantly filled our home and our lives, but after all I had to, because nobody else would.

The boys and I sat down to dinner as darkness fell across the desert. We finished our evening watching television and wrestling before bath time. As I tucked the boys in bed, Jimmy asked, "Mommy, when is daddy coming home?"

"Soon," I answered, kissing him good night. I returned to the living room alone, in the silence that filled the night air. I listened as the pitter patter of soft rain drops started to fall across the roof, imagining they were little angels, parachuting from the heavens.

The television sounded quietly, filling the loneliness with sounds of murmurings, while my thoughts quickly turned back toward the absence of Michael from our lives. I wondered, as I tried to understand how I could compete with an inanimate object, such as a can of beer, or a bottle of Jack Daniels. I hated alcohol, and wondered how I could be so jealous of it! "It is a horrible feeling," I thought, wishing it were another woman. At least I could fend off another woman with violent threats to win him back.

I sat with my legs folded on the sofa, blaming and hating myself for my failures as a wife, and a mother. Why couldn't I stop him from drinking? What was I doing wrong? I wondered if he were with another woman right now, in a bar, kissing her, groping her in a drunken stupor. The visuals formed in my mind and the tears began to flow, as the jealous, bitter emotions, momentarily overcame my love for him. A violent anger, once again, reared its ugly head, enveloping my very existence.

"Why do I even bother to cry over him?" I questioned. It seemed, Michael had become my addiction. Was this possible? Could a woman be addicted a man?

I learned in my adolescent years, the only way to justify my tears, was to be angry. A tear without anger was a form of weakness, which I would not be a part of. As the anger engulfed and swallowed my entire existence, I leapt from the sofa to pace, and weep as I fought back my tears. Nothing would break me because I wouldn't let it! I would fight to the bitter end, even if it took my last breath! I was losing ground to the battle of these great and many, overwhelming fears that would bring about an endless flow of tears, and I knew it.

Suddenly, I remembered going to a Sunday school class, in the small Baptist church I attended as a child. I recalled a teacher telling me how much Jesus loved me, and He would always love me, no matter what happened in life. She said, if I asked Jesus for anything, He would hear, and answer my prayer, because he loved me so much. I knew there was nothing too great, or too hard for Jesus because He was the Son of God. I had nowhere left to run, except to the foot of the cross.

I walked to my bedroom, which was connected through a door in the living room, on the east end of our mobile home. The boys slept quietly in their bedroom that rested at the end of the hall, on the opposite end. Believing Jesus was my last chance, I fell to my knees and folded my hands, resting them on the edge of my bed. This was my last hope. I couldn't take it anymore. The emotional wounds were too deep, and the pain was too great to bear alone. I was helpless. My last hope to stop my pain and sadness, was Jesus. "But, why would He listen to an angry, volatile, downtrodden, worthless woman like me?" I wondered in silence.

As I prayed, audible sobs poured from my throat while I cried out to Jesus, telling Him my story. I shouted His name aloud, "Jesus, help me, please! Save Michael! Make him stop drinking and come home! I need him, and I love him so much! What about our children, Lord? I don't want our children to grow up like me, without a father to love them!" I continued to state my case, telling Him how alone I felt, how our children suffered, and that I couldn't do it by myself. "I need Your help now, Lord Jesus," I begged.

I doubted Jesus' desire to help a simple nobody, a skinny, nothing of a girl like me. I knew I didn't deserve His love, or His help. I loved Jesus, but never really had a relationship with Him, nor did I understand who He really was. I loved Him because I believed that He loved me first and I also believed that He was probably the only one who did. I wondered, wiping my nose across my sleeve, as I violently sobbed and wept, "How could I be sure Jesus would hear me, and do something this time?"

In a last ditch effort, a final desperate plea, a grand finale to get Jesus' attention, I ran to the kitchen and grabbed the largest butcher knife I could find. I didn't really care if I lived or died anymore. I breathlessly gasped for air as I stumbled back to my room, and stood over my bed with the knife in hand.

My heart pounded, and my chin quivered, causing my mouth to twist while I cried out once more, positioning the knife to pierce my heart, "If You really love me, send someone to help me, someone I can talk to, someone who will help me understand. If you really do love me, You will do this for me," I cried, threatening Jesus with my own life.

I pressed the knife into my flesh, slightly twisting it as I woefully swore before God, "I will throw myself down on this knife, and kill myself!" I cried aloud, "I swear I will do it if you don't help me, Lord Jesus. You know my heart! You know I'm not afraid, and You know I will do it," I said, crying out from the depth of my soul. "I would rather be dead than to hurt like this anymore. Hell can't be any worse than my life is!" I had to believe that against all odds, Jesus would take this overwhelming grief from my heart, and deliver us out of our circumstances.

Wiping my eyes and nose once more, I crawled into my bed, and placed the knife under my pillow. A flicker of hope finally prevailed over my tears. I thought, "If I die, someone more able will care for my children. I am all alone, and nobody cares, not even me," I sniveled, drowning in self-pity. "I mean it Lord," I murmured. "I just don't care anymore." I drifted off, nestling my cheek into the damp pillow.

I opened my eyes to a nose pressed into my cheek. Two twinkling blue eyes stared into mine, as Jeffrey lay across me, cupping the sides of my face in his tiny hands. Jimmy, lay across my shoulder, whispering with a small voice in my ear, "Mommy, can we have cereal now?"

I arose with the heaviness of the night before, still looming over me.

Jimmy and Jeffrey dressed themselves to play outside in the sand, still wet from the night's rain. I turned the stereo on, and mused myself in the sunlight as it peeked through the window, warming me. I thought about my prayer and the things I had said to the Lord, the night before. There was a cool breeze flowing into the room from the door, left slightly ajar. I listened for the boys as they played with their Hot Wheels in the cool, damp sand.

Suddenly, I heard a voice whispering something. "What is that?" I mumbled. I turned the stereo off and listened, searching the room to see if someone, or something had crept in, without me noticing. I stood in the stillness of the room, and concluded, I was alone.

I stepped to the center of the living room to listen for the voice again. I heard it again, beckoning me to go to my mother. I thought it to be unsettlingly strange, and very odd that I would hear this. I wasn't sure if I was audibly hearing it, or if I was hearing it in my head, somehow. "Am I crazy? Have I finally, altogether, lost my mind? Am I making this up in my head because I want to go to my mother to seek her sorely needed comfort?"

Again, I heard the soft, faint voice, a little firmer, "Go to your mother!" I found myself arguing, "Oh no, you don't understand! My mother has guests today. She told me she doesn't want me hanging out over there all the time. She will get mad if I go there today." I nervously paced the floor, suspecting it was Jesus, telling me to go to my mother. I don't know how I knew it was Jesus, but somehow, I just knew it was. I heard the same voice, a third time, with a stern, authoritative voice, "Go to your mother, now!"

Like a child who had just received instruction from her father, I walked to the door nervously calling the boys inside. I washed and dressed them in clean clothes and said, "Okay Lord, but if I get in trouble, it's Your fault." With that last word, we walked the short jaunt to my mother's house.

The boy's pushed their way through the gate, running excitedly for grandma's front door. Uncle John and Aunt Lucy had driven out from Monterey Park and I was very excited at seeing them again. We entered the living room, and Aunt Lucy stretched her arms toward the boys for a hug, when the phone rang. My step father, George, answered the phone and said, "Judith, it's for you."

"What?" I said in surprise! "Nobody knows I'm here. Who would be calling me here?" I walked toward the mounted wall phone in the kitchen, keeping an eye on the boys, while lifting the receiver from the table, to my ear. "Hello?" I questioned with a curious voice. Debbie's voice sounded in my ear. Debbie was a friend that was closer than a sister, who lived in Lawndale, an L.A. suburb. Her words resounded, "Hey Judith! You won't believe this, but I have somebody here who wants to talk to you," she giggled. Before I could respond, I heard a male voice come over the phone.

"Hi Judith, please don't hang up! I have some really exciting news I want to share with you," Michael's voice joyously rang through the phone!

After a moment of shocked silence, I exploded into a rage and rebellion that surged through my mind and my heart, all at once. My chin stiffened, as my jaw bore down and locked into position, ready to receive any blow. My thoughts spun into a violent protest with one question after another. "How did he know I was here? Did he really think he could call me, apologize, and return, just like that? How dare he go to my friend's house to call me, and get her to side with, and defend him? How could he do this? How could she do this?" Fighting for composure, and in a hushed voice, I resentfully asked Michael what he wanted. I pulled the phone cord, stretching it to walk into the hallway for privacy. I didn't want to be overheard by the others.

Michael quickly replied, "Judith, I don't blame your for being angry with me. You have every right and I just pray you can forgive me. Something really exciting has happened to me, and I just had to call to tell you about it. I know it's what you always wanted for me," Michael exclaimed gleefully! "I have been born again Judith! I am saved! I have accepted Jesus Christ as my personal Lord and Savior, and yes, I really am….. I am born again!" Michael victoriously continued, "I received the Holy Spirit and the gifts of the Spirit, too. I am saved, Judith! I love the Lord Jesus and I want to come visit. I really miss you guys," he expressed joyfully.

My jaw was no longer locked, and had dropped to my toes. I was stunned and unable to speak. Being the distrusting, wounded woman that I had become, my first thought was, "Oh No! He is not getting out of this one, it won't be that easy for him! One would think, I would have pondered in surprise with thoughts such as; it's a miracle, or He heard me, or He answered my prayer! No, not me. Instead, I thought, "How would I know if he was making this up, or using this as an excuse to come back home." I rejoined our conversation by asking him what he meant by, "Born again."

Michael shared his testimony of being filled with the Holy Spirit and how he was functioning in the gifts of the Spirit. He shared how he had accepted Jesus in his heart, and was born again as a new creature in Christ Jesus. He said the old man, or the old Michael had passed away, proclaiming himself as a new creature. He quoted scriptures he had already memorized such as John 3: 3,

Jesus answered and said to him, "Most assuredly I say to you, unless one is born again, he cannot see the kingdom of God." Jesus answered, "Most assuredly, I say

*to you, unless one is born of water and the Spirit, he
cannot enter the kingdom of God." That which is born of
the flesh is flesh, and that which is born of the Spirit is
spirit.*
And 2 Corinthians 5:17
*Therefore, if anyone is in Christ, he is a new creation;
old things have passed away; behold, all things have
become new.*

After finishing his quotes, he shared his newest
experiences with me. He said the only thing he was sure
about, being new in the Lord, was that he was saved,
received the Holy Spirit and could speak in tongues now.

I defensively embarked on the subject of tongues,
warning Michael not to do that. My mother had told me all
about her Aunt Ollie. She would speak in tongues, dance,
get happy and acted really weird. I warned him, speaking
in tongues was of the devil, and a show for attention. "It's
not of God," I insisted. I cautioned him to be very careful of
what he was getting involved in. Michael snickered at my
comment, making me angrier, if that were possible.

I had known Jesus a lot longer than he had, and I was
the one who had been praying for him. How dare he think
that after being saved for a few days, he already knew
more than me about the bible, and about God? I breathed
out sharply, "You can see the boys if you want to, because
they miss you. You better understand that you and I are
finished and one more thing, if you come to visit us, you
better not do that tongue talking thing in my house!"

"Judith, it is in the bible and when I get there I will
show it to you. We will read the bible together, and I will
tell you all about the gifts of the Spirit," Michael argued
with a gentle, loving voice, unlike I had ever heard him
speak before.

"It is not in the bible," I emphatically argued! I know
I've predominantly read Revelations, and not the rest of
the bible, but I will prove it to you. I will read the New
Testament before you get here and prove it's not in the
King James Bible. You are wrong, Michael. I am not going

45

to sit here and argue with you," I snarled. "Just don't speak tongues in my house, in front of me, or our kids, do you hear me? When are you coming?" I demanded to know.

He said it would be about a week before he could get the gas money, to drive to Cabazon and asked if he could stay on the sofa during his visit. I said it would be alright, as long as he didn't try anything funny. Agitated, and befuddled over the call, I hung up the phone.

Attempting to hide my irritation through a forced smile, I heard my mother ask, "Who was on the phone?"

"Debbie," I responded, still smiling. I didn't dare tell her it was Michael, for fear of seeing the disgust in her expression.

I called the boys to my side to say our brief good byes, and journeyed home.

I sent the boys off to play in their room. Everything felt so surreal. Did Jesus really hear my prayer? Did He really answer me? "I asked You to send someone, Lord, but I didn't expect it to be Michael," I whispered in astonishment! Deep down inside my belly, without understanding, I knew a true miracle of God had just taken place. I was awestruck at what had just happened. I pulled out my bible and read in the book of Matthew. With no idea of what I was doing, I searched the scriptures, reading quickly, and without understanding, I looked for any information to prove there was no such thing as speaking in tongues.

The week carried on as usual. I spent time with the boys, cleaned, and washed the laundry in the bathtub, since we didn't have a washer or dryer. I dug leach lines, worked on septic tanks, and sewed drapes, to earn money locally. With no car to get to town to find work, I took any odd job I could find around Cabazon. In my spare moments, I read my bible, searching for answers. I was nervous about his pending arrival. There was just something so different about him on the phone. My anger was replaced with a warm feeling of expectancy. I knew things were going to be different this time.

I rose early, still nervous and excited about Michael's arrival. The boys were dressed and had breakfast. I dressed, and articulately applied my makeup, to look my best, and make him see what he had lost. Jeffrey smiled his beautiful, dimpled grin, when I told him daddy was coming. Jimmy jumped up and down excitedly with his eyes lit nearly as bright as the sun. The boys were ready to burst in their excitement. I knew I had to stay strong to prevent Michael from taking over, like nothing ever happened. Just then, I heard a car pull up in front of our gate.

Glancing out the window, I saw it was Michael. I hollered, "Daddy's here!" Both boys raced down the hall, aiming for the front door, as I swung it open. They climbed down the three large rail road ties serving as steps, stacked against our three foot high porch. I remained on the porch, watching them run down the path, and lunge into Michael's arms screaming, "Daddy." He glanced up at me, and I saw a new glow in his face. He looked happier, and more confident than I had ever seen him.

Michael spent several hours playing with the boys, while he and I conversed in small talk. Evening approached, and being a gourmet chef, he went into the kitchen to prepare dinner for us. Shortly after dinner, we put the boys to bed early, to give ourselves time together. We settled in the living room, each taking one end of the sofa. We spent the evening discussing his absence, and his drinking. We shared the trials, we each endured during our separation. He said he sat in a bar drinking and feeling guilty for abandoning us, when a man came to witness to him. "I accepted the Lord and it changed my life," he professed. He confessed that he wanted to work things out and become a family again. He suggested we find a church to attend regularly. He knew this was his only salvation from depression, addiction, his past, and the emotional distress that plagued him daily.

During our conversation, we had slowly inched in, moving closer to one another until we sat wrapped in each other's arms. We agreed, everything would work out, now that Jesus Christ was our center. We would be a family again. The night grew dark as our desire for each other grew very passionate.

We entered the bedroom and lay together, upon the bed. Michael moved to lie beside me, and I felt something happen in the very core of my being. Something had exploded inside of me! Oh my God, it was life; I felt it happen, life just exploded in my belly! "I am pregnant," I yelled, sitting up to slap his cheek bone.

Michael jumped with astonishment as my hand struck him, "What was that for," he shouted.

"I'm pregnant," I shouted back. "I told you I wasn't protected. But, no, you said don't worry, I'll be careful."

"What do you mean, you're pregnant? You are not pregnant. How could you know if you are pregnant or not? We just made love! You're crazy, Judith," he scoffed.

"I am pregnant, I just know it. I can't explain, but you'll see, Michael," I said apprehensively, pushing him away from me. I rolled over to turn my back, intent on going to sleep.

Over the course of the next few days, Michael and I found Trinity Broadcasting Network. We watched Christian television and studied our bibles. He shared Acts 2:38,

Then Peter said to them, "Repent, and let every one of you be baptized in the name of Jesus Christ for the remission of sins; and you shall receive the gift of the Holy Spirit.

Along with Acts 10:45,

And those of the circumcision who believed were astonished, as many as came with Peter, because the gift of the Holy Spirit had been poured out on the Gentiles also.

And Mark 16:17,

And these signs will follow those who believe; In My name they will cast out demons; they will speak with new tongues;

As much as I hated admitting I was wrong, I conceded to Michael that tongues were a gift from the Holy Spirit.

Michael laid his hands on me, and prayed. He told me to start moving my tongue and let God do the rest. I was too embarrassed to do it in front of him, and remained unsure whether or not, speaking in tongues was for me. I took my new scriptures and went into the bedroom, closing the door behind me and knelt beside my bed. I asked Jesus to open my heart and show me the truth. "If this is truly a gift from God, let my lips move, and let me begin to speak," I requested. Suddenly, a multitude of new, unfamiliar words, tumbled off the end of my tongue. I felt as if I were soaring through the heavens on the wings of angels! I eagerly ran to Michael, filled to overflowing with a new joy to share my new experience with him.

It had been three months since Michael's return home. I was relieved at having had three menstrual cycles. Albeit, my cycles were irregular, they were not usually regular anyhow. I gave up on the notion of being pregnant, blaming my reaction on my fear of becoming pregnant again. I couldn't imagine myself with three kids and an alcoholic, binging husband. Things were hard enough with two kids. If not for the one abortion I'd had, and several miscarriages, I would be like the old woman in a shoe. I smiled and thanked God for the two children I already had.

We found a wonderful Foursquare Church right behind the Post Office, here in Cabazon. Michael slipped and drank on a couple of occasions, temporarily losing his sobriety. Thankfully, he had not binged for longer than a day, or two. We attended church regularly, and Michael attended A.A. meetings, in his continued battle for life, without alcohol or drugs.

One afternoon, as spring lingered in the air, and the days warmed, I realized how challenging life had become for me. It seemed all I did was worry about when Michael would take his next drink, and where I could hide our money from him this time. I lived in constant fear, on a 24/7 basis. I was leery of falling asleep at night, afraid that when I awoke in the morning hours, he would be gone again. I thought back to the night he returned home, when

I thought I was pregnant, and how frightened I was. I always wanted a little girl. I believed, if we had a little girl, she would be the most beautiful little girl, ever. After much thought, I decided I would be okay with never having that little girl, after all. It would be too difficult for me to manage three children and deal with my husband's addictions, not to mention his constant unemployment. I'm not doing a very good job of keeping our lives together, as it is.

I asked Michael if we could talk about something very serious. I told him how I felt and gave him my take on having more children. "I think it is a bad idea," I said. "As much as I want a girl, I don't need a little girl to fill any voids, or to feel complete, or to be happy. I am happy with our two sons, and I want to get my tubes tied," I explained. "How do you feel?" I asked, carefully examining his face.

"Well," he began, "I wouldn't mind having more kids, but it's okay with me if we don't. Whatever God wants us to do, I guess," he nonchalantly responded.

With what I interpreted as Michael's approval, I walked to my mother's house to call and schedule an appointment for a Tubal Ligation. I explained to the receptionist answering the phone, I had two children and didn't want any more. She scheduled an appointment for me to see Dr. Stanheiser in one week.

I drove to Beaumont to see Dr. Stanheiser alone. I was excited at the prospect of not having to worry about getting pregnant again. It wasn't long before I heard my name called and followed the nurse to a back room. She left me alone, after telling me to disrobe, and handing me a paper gown and a sheet to cover myself with, while I waited for the doctor.

I laid on the examining table, in the cold, drafty, air conditioned room with no clothes, and a thin paper sheet wrapped around me. I pulled the paper sheet against me in an attempt to keep warm. The doctor entered and smiled as she said, "Judith, what are you here for today?"

"I don't want any more children and I hoped, you would tie my tubes for me. I already have two kids, and I really don't want anymore. Gosh, I can barely support the two I have," I giggled.

"Before we do anything, I will have to examine you and run some tests. Take this cup and fill it with a urine specimen. I'll take some blood and we'll do a pap smear. I want to make sure there are no, unforeseen circumstances, or complications that will hinder this. If everything comes back okay, we will proceed from there," she said.

I filled the cup with urine and returned to the examining table. Dr. Stanheiser drew blood and said to lay back and put my feet in the stirrups. I complied and she proceeded with the Pap smear.

"Okay, we are finished here. Go ahead, and get dressed while I take a look at these. I'll be right back.

She returned smiling, as she chuckled with her face lit, announcing, "I think you're a little late for this procedure."

"I don't understand, what do you mean, I'm late? I am confused, I'm not late. My periods have not been normal, but I'm not late. I don't understand what you mean."

She chuckled again and said, "Judith, you are pregnant. I'd say you are about 14 weeks, or so.

"No," I spewed in surprise! "I can't be pregnant! I've had a period every month. I have never had periods during my pregnancies before, never … ever" I bellowed!

I was terrified, "What am I going to do now?" My heart raced, as my worst fear had just become a reality at that very moment in time.

"Everything will turn out okay, Judith," Dr. Stanheiser said, attempting to comfort me. "I know you didn't really want to be pregnant, but you are. You should be happy. We need to schedule you for a follow up exam. Go ahead, and stop at the front desk. They will set an appointment for you next month."

I suddenly became numb, barely able to feel anything. My mind was blank as I stumbled through the parking lot, looking for my car. I drove away feeling a surge of anger manifest, growing stronger with every emotional peak. My mind wandered to thoughts of the night Michael returned home. "I told him I was unprotected, and I was right, I am pregnant! Oh my God! My God, what am I going to do now? I can't do this, God," I screamed aloud! Feeling as if God, were playing some cruel joke on me. I continued to stew on the idea of being pregnant. My anger and resentment toward Michael, and God, grew stronger as I continued home.

I stormed into the living room and immediately ordered the boys to go outside and play, or go to their room. Michael knew by the tone of my voice and the stern look on my face, something had happened. He cocked his head apprehensively, looked up at me from his reclined position and asked, "Are you okay? What's wrong? What happened, Judith?" I saw the alarm in his eyes as he questioned me.

After shutting the front door behind the boys, I yelled, "I'm Pregnant!" I paced across the living room, wanting to throw something. I was so angry!

Michael stood to his feet, and a smile covered his face from ear to hear. He said, "Really?" He raised his arms, as if to praise the Lord, and said, "Aha! It's a girl, I know it's a girl!"

I stopped pacing to stare at him scornfully. I yelled, "You are happy about this? I told you I don't want more children. I am not going to have it," I screamed defiantly, becoming more rebellious, and angrier than I had ever been in my life. "I am making this decision right here and right now, and I will not be persuaded otherwise! You will not change my mind and I will not have another kid period, Michael! Nobody, but nobody will make me have it," I yelled with panicked rage. I stormed in to wash dishes, and before I knew it, dishes were flying all over the kitchen. I screamed, "No God, No, No, No! This can't be happening to me. I will not have another one, I will not, and You can't make me!"

I turned to storm into the bedroom, slamming the door, and I threw my body across the bed, taking a deep breath. I reached over for a cigarette, contemplating how I would get rid of it.

My thoughts were relentlessly pleading with God to end this pregnancy for me. I knew I had to calm down, or I would have a nervous breakdown. I decided I would search for an abortion clinic, tomorrow. I knew Dr. Stanheiser was not going to help me. I also knew, I had to do something fast. If I waited much longer, I would be too far along to get an abortion. I laid across my bed, fighting the feelings of guilt that pursued me in my decision to abort.

"I know Lord, I remember! I remember promising You that I would never have another abortion, but I can't do this.   You just don't understand!" I closed my eyes, recalling the abortion, when I was sixteen years old.

It was early spring, 1973 and I had just moved back home, after having run away from home, rebelling against my life there. There was no love lost between my step father and myself. He was an unhappy, miserable alcoholic and I was a strong willed, rebellious teenager. We fought constantly, yet I still sought his approval and his love, although I never felt I had it. Feeling neglected, shoved aside, and unloved, I sought the attention I so sorely needed from other men who entered my life. While searching for someone to love me, I fell into the seductions of a brief affair with an older man in his mid-thirties, who frequented my step father's garage.

One morning I awoke with severe pain in my left side, and went to the free clinic to be examined. After the examination, the clinician handed me paperwork and said, "I want you to go straight over to the hospital emergency room and take this paper with you. A doctor will examine you there. There is no need for you to return here."

Without question, I blindly did as I was told, handing my paperwork to the front desk. My name was called, and I was escorted to a small examining room. Once again, I disrobed to lay on the examining table, covered by a thin sheet, and waited.

A tall, blond man entered the room, introducing himself, as Dr. Anderson, who would be examining me. I turned my head in embarrassment so I wouldn't look at him in my nakedness that lie open, right in front of him, while he touched me. He finished, informing me that he had found a growth on my left ovary, and I was pregnant.

I felt a chilly numbness come over me, as if my entire body had been injected with lidocaine. I couldn't look at the doctor's face, nor could I speak. In fact, I didn't feel anything at all, except, shame and embarrassment. Every time he asked a question, it was all I could do to nod yes, or no in response. I felt cold, empty and lifeless. Every sound was muted and I was having trouble comprehending my surroundings. When he was finished, I was sent upstairs for a Sonogram, and told to return in two days for my test results.

I left the hospital, afraid and alone, returning home to tell my mother that they had found a growth on my ovary, and I was pregnant. Once I entered the safety of my mother's presence, I felt protected and secure again. It was the kind of protection that only my mother could offer me. I sat on the sofa next to the recliner, where my mother relaxed watching television. I was afraid to tell her I was pregnant, and so, I started with my medical condition first. I told her I had a growth on my ovary, and quickly blurted, "And I'm pregnant," discarding any emotion, and as a matter of fact. I continued "I'm scared, and don't know what to do," I confided. I didn't want her to know, just how scared I really was. The tension grew while I waited for her response. After a very long, silent moment, I told her I had to return in two days, to get my test results.

She remained silent in her recliner, listening to me.

"Maybe she isn't mad at me after all," I thought.

There it was! I looked into her eyes searching for her comfort, and instead, I saw the hardness of her fury settling in her expression as her eyebrow lifted. She shook her head with her lips pursed tight, closing her hands to make a fist, with only the index finger of her right hand, pointing toward the floor.

Barely parting her lips to speak, her firm voice rang out to scold me. "If you have this child, you will have to go on welfare and live on the streets, because I will not have another child in my house to take care of." She continued, "I don't want another baby, on along someone else's baby to take care of. I have six children! Don't you think I have enough responsibilities without you running out and getting pregnant?" she reviled. Then her shocking words blindsided me,

"You had better get an abortion, Judith Ann! Think about it, you don't have a choice. You can't take care of it! You will have to live on the streets by yourself. You don't have any money, or a job, or a house, and you haven't even finished high school. What are you going to do with a baby, young lady? You have nearly embarrassed me right out of town," her words seethed from between her lips.

"I don't want you to tell anyone about this! Nobody! Do you understand me, Judith? Nobody, nobody, nobody….. or we will pack up and move back to Cabazon, leaving you here to live on the streets with that baby, all alone," she said, threatening me into obedience. It seemed my mother had never even heard me tell her about the growth on my ovary.

I was more afraid and ashamed than ever, knowing I had embarrassed and shamed my own mother. I could never tell anyone who the father was without risking his arrest for statutory rape. I suddenly understood, how alone I really was. I thought about my mother's words, and I knew she was right. How was I going to care for this child, or provide for it? The idea of living on the streets with a baby scared the hell right out of me. It was right then, I shut down, again. I couldn't feel anything, I couldn't think, and I didn't want to think anymore. I was too scared! I decided to do what my mother had told me to do, abort the baby and put it all behind me. I would just do it, and I wouldn't think about it anymore.

Two days later, my mother drove me back to the county hospital, dropping me off on the far side of the parking lot. She was embarrassed and didn't want anyone to see her with me. I got out of the car and watched my mother drive away as I walked across the large parking lot to the entrance. I took a deep breath before going in, afraid and all alone, I knew I had to do this alone. I returned to the window located next to the ER, and waited for several hours, before my name was called. I was led to a room in the back, handed a cloth gown and sheet, and told, "You know the routine, undress." I undressed and waited for the doctor to return.

The doctor entered, and introduced himself once more, as though he thought I had forgotten. He asked how I was feeling and I turned my head to avoid looking, or speaking to him. I was too embarrassed and ashamed to speak to anyone. In the middle of the examination, he asked if I wanted this pregnancy. I shook my head to signal, "No," and he assertively responded, "Okay, don't worry, I'll take care of it for you." I wasn't quite sure what he meant by, "I'll take care of it for you," and was too afraid to ask. I assumed it meant he was going to do the abortion. When he was finished, I was told to get dressed and meet him across the hall, in his office.

I tapped on the large white door that held a modest brown label, with "Dr. Anderson" inscribed across it. I heard a voice call, "Come in." I entered to see the doctor writing notes. There were two small padded chairs in front of his desk, and he gestured for me to take a seat. I sat as he lifted his eyes toward me, and asked, "Do you have any questions for me?"

I looked over his desk to avoid eye contact. I was numb and so stiff that I could barely move. I listened to every word he spoke and was unable to find my own words, all I could do was nod my head.

Dr. Anderson seemed to be genuinely concerned, telling me, he had found a lump on my ovary two days ago. He said two days ago it was about the size of a grape and today's exam revealed the lump had grown to the size of his fist. He was concerned that if the lump continued to grow at this rate, it may rupture, causing other complications.

He told me, he would open me up in surgery to remove the mass, but they would not close the incision until after they received the biopsy results. If there was any form of cancer, or any other threatening disease, he would perform a radical hysterectomy. He told me it was in my best interest to have an abortion since the fetus had been subjected to harmful amounts of radiation through testing, and it may cause deformities. He asked if I clearly understood what he had told me. Again, I nodded my head, yes.

He told me there was no time to waste and wanted to hospitalize me immediately. He would run tests this afternoon and operate first thing in the morning. He asked, "Are you afraid? Do you realize how serious this is, Judith?"

I finally got enough nerve to speak and said, "Why should I be afraid? Isn't it minor surgery? In and out?" I asked, staring past him. I wasn't about to let anyone know how scared I really was.

"No Judith, this is not a simple surgery. This is a very serious health issue and it is a major surgery that I will be performing on you tomorrow!" He asked again, "Are you sure you don't have any questions for me?"

I silently shook my head,"No."

"Okay then, go get checked in, and I will see you in the morning," he said, dismissing me.

I slowly paced myself as I walked to admissions, searching for a pay phone along the way. I found one and inserted a dime to tell my mother I wouldn't be coming home.

"Hello?"

"Hi mom," I said. I continued to tell her that the doctor would abort the pregnancy, and I was immediately being admitted to the hospital. I explained that I was having a major surgery, and would be in the hospital for about a week.

"Everything will be fine, just remember to be strong," and call me when you're released. I'll pick you up."

I hung up and proceeded to the registration window.

After I was taken to my room, different technicians came in and out, running tests in preparation for surgery. After a short rest, a team of eight interns entered my room with Dr. Anderson. The doctor stood before the group of men, all standing at the end of my bed. He discussed my medical condition, and pending surgery in medical terms, most of which I didn't understand. When he was finished, each intern took his turn spreading my legs and inserting their fingers inside of me. I was horrified by all the male interns looking at me, touching me. I felt as if I were being gang raped. I stared at the wall, refusing to look up, or acknowledge the men in my grave humiliation.

Evening fell and my eye lids became heavy. Before long, I drifted off to sleep.

I awoke that morning to a nurse injecting a needle into my hip and saying I may become sleepy. I struggled to stay awake, but in no time, I succumbed to the drug meant to relax me, and fell asleep.

A bright light shone on me and I could faintly hear voices. I didn't know where I was, or who the people were that surrounded me. I had a strong urge to urinate and attempted to raise myself up, finding it quite difficult to raise my body. I heard a shout and suddenly, people were grabbing my arms from both sides. A stern voice ordered me to lay down and be still. I didn't know where I was or why these people were hollering and grabbing me.

"I have to go to the bathroom," I cried aloud. "Please let go of me, I have to go pee!" I struggled to free my arms when I heard a familiar voice call my name. Dr. Anderson said I had a catheter in place, and would feel the urge to urinate. He assured me, I wasn't going to wet myself.

"Okay," I murmured, laying my head back down as darkness fell over me once again.

I awoke in Recovery to the severe pain in my belly. I searched for a call button to get something for the pain. I struggled to raise myself from the bed, while lifting the bandage to see where they had cut me horizontally from hip to hip. There were small black stitches along the incision, stained with Betadine. The nurse came in and I told her that it hurt. She gave me a shot and handed me a nightgown and robe that had been dropped off by my mother at the nurse's station. I asked where my mother was, and was told that she had dropped by after the surgery, and quickly left. I was afraid and longed for the security of my mother's love and protection and was disappointed at missing her. The pain shot kicked in, causing me to close my eyes, as I drifted off.

I awoke the following morning to Dr. Anderson asking me how I felt. "It hurts," I told him. He said the abortion was successful, and the biopsy showed the tumor to be benign cancer. He said he removed my appendix as a precaution, and everything else was still intact. He asked if I had any questions. Half asleep, I shook my head no and he left the room. Lunch came and went and I laid in bed watching television. I developed Bronchitis while in the hospital and coughed hard enough to rip open one end of my incision. Watching a program on television, I heard someone mention cancer. Suddenly, it hit me, Dr. Anderson said I had some kind of cancer. I couldn't remember the word he used. I was very frightened and trembled at the thought of dying.

I had to call my mother. I had no idea what kind of cancer it was. I put on my robe, and struggled to raise myself from the bed. Waves of excruciating pain shot through my belly and my back. I used the I.V. pole to steady myself and assist me down the long corridor, leading to the pay phones. Every step I took shot another excruciating pain through my belly. The waiting room at the end of the corridor was full. A gentleman pushed his chair over to me as I reached for the phone receiver, still using the I.V. pole to hold myself up. I thanked him, sat down and dialed my mother's number.

Trishly, my younger sister, answered the phone. I asked for mom and she replied, "Mom isn't here, she's next door." I told her I was at the hospital and it was really important. I asked her to run as fast as she could to get mom and bring her to the phone. A couple of minutes had passed before I heard my mother breathlessly whisper, "Hello."

I burst into tears at the sound of her voice, and proceeded to tell her I had some kind of cancer, as I sobbed uncontrollably.

"What kind of cancer is it," my mother asked. I told her I couldn't remember the word the doctor used. I had never heard the word before.

"I will talk to the doctor right now," she responded and hung up the phone.

I returned to my room where I laid sobbing in my bed. I was only sixteen years old and I was going to die. How could I have cancer? My eyes swelled and my head pounded from crying so hard.

A couple of hours passed before my mother came in and stood at the foot of my bed, as though she were afraid to get too close to me. "The doctor said the tumor was benign, which means no cancer. Benign means no cancer was found, Judith." Just then the nurse came in and said the doctor ordered a sedative to help you sleep. My mother, told me she couldn't stay and said I'd be fine. I cried after her as she walked away, leaving me alone in my hospital bed. I turned my eyes toward the window feeling abandoned and alone, drifting off to sleep.

The next morning, the father of my aborted child stopped by to thank me for having the abortion, and for not telling anyone about us as he quickly turned to leave. He was my only visitor since my pregnancy was top secret, and nobody could know that I was here.

Five days sped by quickly and Dr. Anderson released me. I called my mother to pick me up and met her in the parking lot.

I sat on the sofa, took a pain pill and sighed, "Home at last." It was finally over.

The medication did its job as long as I sat still. My head was foggy and every sound echoed around me, until I could no longer think clearly. It was the pain pills. My mind wandered in the fog as I recalled the events of the last couple of weeks. I thought about my hospital stay and the prior doctor visits.

I remembered the doctor asking me if I wanted the pregnancy. I wondered how he could have, so flagrantly told me, he would take care of it without any emotion or feeling. Didn't he know he was about to kill a little baby? He called the baby an, "It." "It," was a baby. It was my baby.

Oh my God! I suddenly realized, I just killed a baby..... I killed my own baby! For the first time since all this began, my mind was clear, and I realized with a complete accounting of what I had done. The consciousness that I had murdered my own child, struck me like a brick upside my head.

The Ten Commandments raced through my mind, and self-condemnation tore at my heart. "Oh Jesus, I have committed murder! What am I going to do? What is going to happen to me? Am I going to hell now?" I thought quietly. My thoughts raged violently in my mind and the guilt ripped through my heart. A sudden fear came over me and I struggled to stand to my feet. I grabbed my purse and started for the door.

"Where are you going?" my mother asked.

"I'm walking to the corner to get a pack of cigarettes," I answered, walking out the front door. I ambled toward the market where I had seen a pay phone. I fought desperately to hold back the tears as images of murdering my baby and the flames of hell clouded my mind, consuming every bit of me. I couldn't hold back the tears anymore. As they broke through one by one, flowing from my eyes and over my cheeks, I held my head up and kept walking. I had to get to the phone to call my cousin, Richard. The only number I knew was my Aunt Lucy's. I could only hope he would be there. Richard was an ordained Minister of God, and I believed he was the only one who could help me, and keep my secret confident. We had been very close growing up. I had to find him to tell him what I had done and beg him to pray for me.

I finally reached the pay phone and dialed "0" for the operator. I placed a collect call to Aunt Lucy's phone, and listened as she accepted charges. Her voice came over the phone, "Judith? Judith, what is wrong?" She listened to me sniffle and sob. "Aunt Lucy, I have to talk to Richard," my voice crumbled in my brokenness. I was undone. I violently cried and she struggled to understand my fragmented words. She said Richard wasn't there, but if I gave her a phone number she would have him call me right back. I gave her the phone number and hung up, keeping my hand gripped tightly on the receiver.

A couple of minutes passed before the pay phone rang. I lifted the receiver to my ear and cried out Richard's name. I sobbed and confessed to murdering my own baby. I said I was going to hell. He calmly told me about the forgiving grace, and endless mercies of our Lord Jesus Christ. He tried to convince me I wouldn't go to hell because I was repentant. He said he could hear how sorry I was for what I had done. Richard prayed with me, comforted me, and encouraged me to stop crying. I told him how much I loved him and thanked him, begging him not to tell anyone about our conversation. I hung up, and left to find a place to be alone with God.

I hid in the nearby alley, where I conversed with Jesus. I repented, telling Him how sorry I was, and how much I hated myself for what I had done. "You may forgive me, Jesus, but I don't think I can ever forgive myself." I didn't deserve to live after murdering an innocent baby, on along murdering my own baby. "How could I have done this?" I wondered. The tears streamed down my face as my heart raged against me, making me wish I were dead for what I had done. My heart cried out to Jesus and I promised Him, no matter what happens, I will never do anything like this again. I will never have another abortion, or murder another child again! I pleaded with Jesus to stop me, if I ever tried to something like this again. I asked Him to do whatever He had to, to stop me! "Please Jesus, don't ever let me do this again," I cried aloud in desperation, wiping my eyes as I stood up, took a deep breath and slowly started for home.

I heard a creaking noise, coming from my bedroom door as Michael opened it, jarring me out of the emotional memories of my past, and back to reality. He came into the room and sat next to me on the bed.

"Are you hungry?" he gently asked. I have dinner ready. It's on the table and the boys and I are waiting for you."

"I'll be right there," I said. I went into the bathroom to splash some water on my face. I was a little shaken after recalling the memories of the abortion I'd had so many years ago. It didn't matter anymore. I couldn't have another child and God and Michael would just have to understand that.

We cleaned up the kitchen and put the boys to bed while we spent the evening together in prayer, and discussed my pregnancy. I told Michael I had made up my mind and I was going to have an abortion. I vowed, nobody would stop me. I just couldn't bear having another child. Things were difficult enough, as it was. I could see by the countenance of Michael's face, he was very saddened by my declaration of the necessity for an abortion. He decided to leave it in prayer, putting it in God's hands.

Michael stayed up to read his bible, and pray, while I retired for the evening. I slipped on my nightgown, curled up in the bed, and snuggled into the blankets to get warm. My mind wandered through the corridors of guilt, filling my heart as I convinced myself that I was going to abort this pregnancy. I tried to push the thoughts and visions of a dead baby out of my mind. I closed my eyes and drifted off into a twilight slumber.

I heard a voice calling out to wake me, "Judith!" The voice I heard echoed in my conscience mind, assaulting me back to my regrets of abortion once again. The remorse swept over me as I closed my eyes, pushing my feelings aside, and once more, drifted off to sleep.

It seemed only moments had passed before I got up from my bed with excruciating pain rising up and down along my back. The tears began to flow as the pain overwhelmed my already exhausted body. I walked into the bathroom and noticed a small amount of blood on the back of my nightgown. I cleaned myself up, not knowing why I had this terrible pain, or what was causing it. I decided it was best to drive myself to the hospital. As I entered in through the emergency room doors, a nurse, seeing the abundance of blood, ran to my aid. I saw the blood begin to flow from between my legs and cried out, "Oh my God!".....

Chapter 3
EMOTIONALLY ABORTED

The nurse had not wasted any time, seeing the abundance of blood, covering my nightgown. The blood flowed down my inner thighs, as I doubled over with the pain that wrenched against my belly. She laid me on to a gurney, pushing me down a long corridor. I felt dizzy, disoriented, and unaware of my surroundings. We entered a room at the end of the corridor and she pushed the gurney over to the bed that stood in the center of the small room. With great difficulty and assistance, I climbed on to the bed and laid back. The nurse grabbed my legs and placed them into the stirrups. I gazed around the room, pressing my fists into my lower abdomen in an attempt to ease the pain, realizing I was in a delivery room. Violence apprehended my mind when I saw my blood covering the floor of the delivery room. I screamed in horror, watching the faceless nurse wield a large knife, slashing my baby to death. The blood on the floor was not mine, but the life of my child, draining from its limp body. "Stop," I shrieked in horror, "STOP, STOP … STOP IT!"

"Judith, Judith!" I stirred hearing a voice call my name, and gently shaking me. I gasped for air with trembling hands, while my mind spun and grappled for a visual that wasn't so terrifying. "Judith, you're dreaming, wake up," he said, leaning over to look at me as I struggled for some remnant of sanity.

I slowly stretched my neck to see the sun peeking through the gaps in the curtain, covering the small window over our bed and realized it was all a nightmare.

"I guess I was dreaming," I smiled at him and shook off the memory of that terrifying nightmare.

After breakfast, Michael drove to town, and returned to announce that he was the new chef at a small dinner house.

He excitedly suggested a picnic at the park to celebrate his new found employment. I made my excuses so I could find an abortion clinic. I offered to make a picnic basket and urged them to go without me. "It'll be fun for the boys," I announced. Michael left with Jimmy and Jeffrey for a boy's day out.

I begged God to take this pregnancy from me so I wouldn't have to have an abortion. I couldn't bear the thought of another child depending on me. What if Michael drank again? What if he took off, abandoning us again? I was betraying Jesus by breaking my promise to never have another abortion. I repeatedly told Him I was sorry. I knew beyond any shadow of doubt, I could not, and would not take on the responsibility of one more life!

After praying, I borrowed my mother's phone book, and located an abortion clinic in Riverside. I spoke with a woman who confirmed, they would terminate the pregnancy for me. I scheduled an appointment for the following week.

After hanging up the phone, I joined my mother in the living room, where she watched her soap operas. I attempted a conversation with her, but she was wrapped up in the soaps, so I left for home.

Michael, and the boys returned home from the park later that afternoon. After they settled in, I told Michael I had made an appointment next week for an abortion. We argued and snarled at each other and I reaffirmed, I had made up my mind. I told him I needed the car that day. I would drive him to work, but he would have to find another ride home, and I would be back home the same day. In his disappointment, he walked into the kitchen and began praying.

My mind was fretfully set on my to-do-list before tomorrow's appointment at the clinic. After Michael left for work, I finished my morning chores and walked to Sylvia's house with the boys. Sylvia was my brother Daryl's, girlfriend and lived around the corner from us. We both had sons around the same age and quickly became friends. She had agreed to watch Jimmy and Jeffrey when I went in to have the abortion procedure.

"I pray every day asking, no, begging God to take this pregnancy from me," I confided to Sylvia. She listened quietly, assuring me that everything would turn out for the best. I wasn't sure Sylvia agreed with what I was doing, but she knew I would neither be hindered, nor stopped. I was confident that everything was going as planned.

It was nearly time for Michael to return from work. "C'mon boys, Jimmy… Jeffrey, let's go!" I called out. "It's time to go home now. Daddy will be home shortly."

We met Michael at the gate, arriving home at the same time. I left the boys with him and took the car to gas up, before returning home to make dinner. It took the last of our money to fill the tank with gasoline for the eighty mile round trip to Riverside.

Michael had already started dinner when I returned. I joined him in the kitchen to fry some potatoes and warm a can of pork beans. We added hot dogs, onions, and various spices to make dinner a little more interesting.

As the evening progressed, Michael made one last attempt to talk me out of the abortion. "Maybe God gave us this child, Judith. I can't make you do anything, but I want you to know I don't want you to do this. Please, Judith, don't do this. God does not approve," he pleaded desperately in a hushed, yet stern voice.

I immediately jumped to my own defense, blaming him for what I was about to do. "If you had just waited for me to get birth control, this wouldn't be happening at all. Do you really think this is what I wanted? Just leave me alone, Michael! I will not have another kid," I defiantly yelled. My mind was made up and nothing would stop me. I crawled into bed and closed my eyes in an attempt to shut out Michael's words, and prayed.

"If you don't take this pregnancy from me, Lord, I will have to abort it. Don't you understand, I can't do this? Michael is still drinking. I can't have another child. I won't! Please God, don't make me do this. I can't even properly feed or care for the two I have. I feel so guilty Lord, but I have to do it. Michael only works part time and there is not enough work to supply all of our needs," I cried, begging Jesus to hear and answer me. Guilt, anger and fear overcame my emotions as I realized that Jesus, and Michael were both disappointed in me. I knew God was sending me to hell, but this was what I had to do.

I decided I was more afraid of having another child than I was of going to hell. Besides, God couldn't hurt me any worse than I was already hurting. "Why was God so cruel? He is a mean God," I thought. "He is always ready to send me to hell at any given opportunity. But Jesus, well, at least Jesus loves me. He will forgive me and understand."

"Now, I will give God plenty of reasons to send me to hell. How much more could He do to me?" I was determined to follow through with my plan to abort.

I lifted my head from the thin, worn pillow to look at the clock. The alarm was about to sound any minute. I got an early jump on the shower while Michael got ready for work. We didn't speak to one another as we prepared for the day ahead. "Okay, Jimmy, Jeffrey, let's go, we have to take daddy to work," I shouted.

We drove Michael to work for his early 7 a.m. start. My appointment was at 10 a.m., leaving me with plenty of time to meet both deadlines. Everyone was very quiet as we rode to Banning. The boys sat in the back seat watching out the windows, sensing the tension and remained very still. An eerie sense of fear and uncertainty clouded the atmosphere around us. The tension was very thick. Determination was driving at my heart in fierce rebellion against God, Michael, or anyone else who would try to stop me from having this abortion. I was unwaveringly determined, and nothing was going to stop me!

The boys and I returned home to turn on cartoons and entertain them as I took out my bible. I couldn't bring myself to open and read the pages that I knew would convict my heart. I wasn't going to let anything persuade me, or get in the way, not even God!

"I'm sorry, Jesus," I whimpered, praying again. "I love You, but You just don't understand. I asked You to take this child so I wouldn't have to do this. I know in my heart You want me to have this baby and I know Michael wants it too, but I don't. I can't, I'm too afraid. Don't You get it? I don't want another child! I can't take any more heartaches, or struggles. My life is too difficult as it is and I am already overburdened with more than I can handle. Can't You see how it hurts me, or how afraid I am? Why have You done this and why won't You take this child from me? You can fix it so that I won't have to do this. Please….," my voice trailed into a whisper begging God in this, my final moment.

It was time to get started. "Jimmy….. Jeffrey, it's time to go. C'mon and I'll take you to Sylvia's. You can play with your friends while mommy goes to town." The boy's ran into the living room to grab a toy, completely unaware of what was about to happen. "I'll pick you up when daddy gets home from work," I announced, preparing to leave.

"Get in the car now," my voice elevated as they lollygagged. The boys climbed into the back seat and I slid in behind the wheel of the car. I took a deep breath and once again I said, "I'm sorry, Jesus!" I inserted the key into the ignition and turned it to start the engine.

"What?" I gasped in surprise, and my hand slapped the steering wheel. Agitated and frustrated, I yelled for the boys to be quiet as they teased and played with each other in the back seat. I turned the key back toward the "Off" position, and turned it again. Nothing, not even a click sounded. Again, I turned the key, and nothing, not a click, or a ping, nothing at all. Dead silence rung against my ears in the stillness of the rising temperatures in this forsaken desert land.

"No, No, NOOOOO!" I screamed as my fist pounded against the steering wheel, "NO!!!" I got out of the car and heatedly said, "No problem, I'll fix it." After all, I had worked on a lot of cars over the years in the garage with my step-father and on my own cars too. I prided myself in knowing more about cars than the average man. It had to be the battery, alternator, or starter. "Why wouldn't it start," I wondered, lifting the hood.

I noted there was no corrosion on the battery. The battery fluid checked out okay and I was getting spark from the battery. The alternator and ignition were firing and seemed fine.

"Oh no! What am I going to do?" I threw my hands up, shaking my head in desperation.

We quickly walked to Sylvia's house. She saw how upset I was and asked, "What's wrong?"

"Can you give me a ride to Riverside?" I asked wildly panicked. "My car wouldn't start. I don't understand, I just used it to take Michael to work this morning. Now, when I turn the key there is nothing at all. It's just dead!" I begged her from the bowels of my desperation, to take me to the clinic in Riverside.

"I don't have any gas in my car, but if you have gas money, then, I guess I could take you," Sylvia replied.

"I don't have any money left at all. Don't you know anyone you could borrow the money from? I'll pay you back when Michael gets paid, please," I urgently pressed her.

"No, I don't know anyone who isn't broke," she replied.

"Okay, I'll have to reschedule for next week. Will you drive me to Riverside next week if I can reschedule for then, and take care of the boys? I will fill your tank and babysit for you when I'm feeling better," I offered hostilely.

"I'll drive you there," she calmly promised. "You just have to put gas in my car."

"I'm sorry, I'm going home because I am too angry right now. I'll see if my step father will look at my car and see what's wrong with it," I stated in utter disgust and left.

I ordered the boys to their room, warning them to leave me alone for a while. I had not anticipated the car not starting. Our 1970 Mercury Montego had been running just fine. There were no warnings to let me know the car was about to break down. "I just don't understand it," I murmured aloud.

"Okay God, this is not funny. I am really angry!" I said, with a threatening tone. "You are not going to stop me! I will find a way," I blatantly declared!

"Boys, it's time to walk to grandmas," I said, pulling them by my side as I locked the door. My mother was at work in a nearby truck stop, where she was being promoted to manager and my step father was out and about. I went inside and sat the boys down in front of the television while I called the clinic.

After apologizing, I explained to the receptionist that my car wouldn't start and rescheduled in another week. I assured her, this time I would be there. Next, I called Michael at work to tell him the car wouldn't start, causing me to miss my appointment. I quickly became annoyed with him while detecting a hint a joy in his voice at missing my appointment. He wasn't even upset about the car. I told him he would have to find his own way home and that I had rescheduled for next week.

We walked outside to leave when my step father drove up. He grabbed a bag of groceries and walked to the garage. I followed, telling him what had happened to my car. He was the kingpin of mechanics and there was nothing he didn't know about cars. I was confident he would be able to fix it, or at least diagnose the problem for me. When I finished, he stood with his hands in his pockets and stared at the ground deep in thought. After a moment, he said, "Michael will be home soon. He will figure it out. If he can't, then I'll take a look at it." With that answer, I grabbed the boys and returned home.

I made lunch and returned to look at the car once more. I turned the key in the ignition, and nothing. I was absolutely bewildered and didn't understand why the car wouldn't start. I returned inside, frustrated and fatigued. I laid on the sofa to rest while the boys played together after lunch.

Michael came home early to see what he could do about getting the car running again. He was unusually cheerful, especially after a hot day in the kitchen. He asked for more details about the car and seemed disinterested in talking about my missed appointment. I was irritated at his indifference. He needed the car for work and I understood that, but I still felt neglected. I described the car's symptoms along with my anger at missing my appointment. Michael lifted his head and said, "I don't understand it either, there wasn't any warning. I'll check it out," he said, walking out the front door.

I raised to follow him to the car. I watched as he opened the driver's door, slid in and inserted the key into the ignition. He sat very still for a moment, lowered his head as if to have a word with God, and turned the key. Instantly, the engine fired right up without hesitation. Michael sat there with a grin on his face and glanced up at me. "There doesn't seem to be anything wrong with it. It started right up for me," he smirked.

For a moment, I felt like a foolish child, caught in a lie. "Well, it wouldn't start for me," I sassed back! Confused, I ran back into the house, "Okay, what just happened here?" I sat on the sofa stewing in the bubbling juices of my own self-righteous indignation

"Oh no, You did not do this, God! I won't let You get away with this," I declared as I laughed aloud in the face of God. "I already have a ride next week and nobody is going to stop me. NOT EVEN YOU, GOD!" I looked upward, toward Heaven, and vowed, "I WON'T HAVE THIS BABY!"

With a strong dedication to my own "Will Power," I stomped into the kitchen engulfed in anger. It was my will to "not," have this child and I wasn't going to have it. As I tried to forget the day, I slammed dishes and threw food against the counter as I started preparing dinner. Dinner wouldn't take long since all we had left were a couple of boxes of macaroni and cheese. I set the table and Michael called the boys in. I stabbed every noodle with the prongs of my fork as if it were my enemy. After a few bites, I went to my room to be alone and sulk.

The week had passed and I was feeling jittery about my appointment in Riverside, tomorrow. I walked to Sylvia's and asked her to start her car. I needed to know it would start so I could rest. We walked to her car and I watched as she turned the key. The engine fired up without any hesitation. I returned home, comfortable that it would all work out.

Michael avoided bringing up the subject of abortion. He knew how angry it made me, but not without first making it known he was against it. He continued to pray God's will be done, and not ours. I lay on my bed and asked Jesus why He wouldn't help me. I didn't want to have an abortion, but I felt that God was forcing my hand. I set my alarm and struggled to fall asleep. After several hours of mental anguish and fighting with God, I finally drifted into a twilight sleep, a half sleep, half-awake slumber, never feeling like I was ever asleep.

The radio alarm blared in my ear as morning arrived. Michael left for work and I fed the boys breakfast. They watched cartoons while I apprehensively watched the clock from the edge of my seat.

I was well into my second trimester and running out of time. This had to happen today, or I would be too far along to do it.

I was very emotionally charged with anticipation, as we walked to Sylvia's house. The boys ran off to play in the back room while Sylvia finished dressing.

The six of us walked to Sylvia's car to begin the day's journey. We loaded the kids, toys, and packed lunches into the car. Sylvia and I slid into the front seats and adjusted ourselves for the long drive. She slipped the key into the ignition and turned the key.

"Uh-Oh," Sylvia croaked, glancing up at my face. I looked up to see her turning the key back and forth. There was nothing, not even a click. The car was dead. Sylvia was as dumbfounded as I was. My jaw dropped. I stared at her dashboard looking for lights, or any sign of life in her car.

This could not be happening again! This was not coincidence. This was God! How dare He do this to me again! I opened the car door, stepped out into the dirt and ordered the boys to get out of the car. I leaned over to Sylvia, "If you get it started, please come and get me. I'm going home," I angrily announced. With a sick, dead feeling in my gut, I reached out to grab the boys and their things, and began my journey home.

My legs were numb along with the rest of me. The anger built up inside of me with every lengthy step my long, slender legs stretched to. Anger was now my drug of choice. My rage was so strong, it made me feel invincible, nearly immortal and nothing could hurt me anymore. My rage was my determination, my fuel, my strength, and nothing could take me down, or stop me now!

I looked to make sure Jimmy and Jeffrey were still beside me with their short, little legs running to keep up with me. I turned and yelled, "You better hurry up," as I verbally accused and argued aloud with God. "Why God?" I disdainfully asked. "Why? Why are You doing this to me? You don't care about me," I continued, "You know how I feel. You know I don't want another kid. Why are you making me have it? I don't want it and I won't have it. Stop this, God, Stop it!" I snapped, as ire fueled the adrenaline that rushed through my body.

I grabbed Jimmy and Jeffrey as I unlocked the door and guided them inside and they ran straight to the television to turn on cartoons. I paced back and forth until I had gone beyond angry. I became incensed, yes, incensed beyond measure. I stopped in the middle of the room, exasperated in a fury of rebellion and rage. The ferocity of this furious antagonism was a new experience for me. The strength I felt in it made me think that I was foolishly unconquerable, as though nobody, or nothing could defeat me. I wanted to scream at the top of my lungs. I held back, knowing that once I started to scream, I wouldn't be able to stop.

Without warning, I suddenly heard a voice screaming. It was brash, defiant and obnoxious. It was my voice, as I screamed and looked upward. My finger pointed toward God in heaven and I began to swear at Him. I could no longer control my voice, my thoughts, or my emotions. Rage had taken over and there was no stopping it now! The voice that came out of me was a wrath filled, rebellious defiance toward God, and I began to shout even louder.....

"Just who do you think you are, God? You can't do this to me, You don't have the right! I won't let You! You won't get away with this, do You hear me? I will not have this baby, and You are not big enough to make me have it,"

I growled as I slowly and methodically enunciated every word in a clear, concise, threatening tone. I swayed forward and backward, with one leg extended outward, and slightly bent at the knee, thrusting my finger back and forth at Him, screaming as loud as I could, making sure He heard every word.

"I will not have this child and You can't make me! I hate You God, I hate You! You are not so big and tough, or so powerful that You can stop me from aborting this pregnancy. I will not have this baby, God, I will not. I will fight You! Come down here, NOW! I will fight You and I will not lose this battle! Do You hear me? Do you hear me, God? I will fight You!"

I bellowed in a bold challenge against the one and only, "Almighty God!"

I turned to change my position to a fighting stance and drew back my fist, when from the corner of my eye, I saw an unnatural movement.

I turned to see a flame flickering in the window. Fire! There was a fire outside of my living room window. In that one small flicker, I went from "irate", to "protect." I yelled, "Jimmy … Jeffrey!" I continued to yell their names while running through the house in search of them.

I ran down the long hall to their bedroom, and found Jimmy hiding in the closet. "Come here, Jimmy," I demanded. I pulled him into the living room and asked, "Where is your brother?" He was afraid to answer me because of all my yelling. I drug him through the house by his arm, calling Jeffrey's name repeatedly. Panicked, I asked him again, "Where is your brother, where did he go?" Jimmy shrugged, an "I don't know." I squeezed into the corner to look behind the sofa, and saw a little foot. There was Jeffrey, tucked away, hiding behind the sofa. I reached in and grabbed him, then Jimmy and ran out the door. I took the boys across the street to a neighbor we called, Granny. "I don't have a phone, Granny. Would you call the fire department for me?"

I left the boys in her care and ran back inside to look out the window again, to be sure of the fire. We lived in a two bedroom mobile home on a double lot enclosed with a six foot, wooden fence. Our Back yard was also enclosed on either end by the six foot wood fence, butting against the walls of our mobile home. It appeared that the fence in our back yard is where the fire began. I watched as the tips of the flames were stretching, reaching out for the walls of my home. I knew I didn't have much time to put the fire out before it overtook and burned our home, along with all of our possessions. I thought about Jimmy and Jeffrey's baby books, photo albums, and our clothes, these were about all the treasures we owned. We were about to lose it all. I was going to have to fight to save our home.

I wished Michael was here to help me. "Oh my God," I exclaimed! "I'm sorry, God, I'm so sorry, I didn't mean it," I howled, engulfed with fear and forgetting all about my anger.

I ran back outside, lifted the hose and reached for the water spigot to turn it on. As I reached for the spigot, I remembered we had removed it to prevent the boys from playing in the water. I ran back inside, pulling open the kitchen junk drawer. I tossed the items in the drawer in search of the spigot handle. It wasn't there! I pulled the drawer completely out and dumped it on the floor. It wasn't there. I pulled out the second junk drawer to get the pliers. I frantically continued to pull out every drawer in the kitchen, ransacking each one in search of the pliers. They were nowhere to be found.

Pandemonium and dread overtook my senses as I ran out the gate and back to Granny's. "Do you have any pliers, Granny? I can't find mine and I need them to turn my water hose on." Granny shook her head, "No."

I grabbed Jimmy by the shoulders and turned him to face me. "Jimmy, do you think you can find your way to Grandma's house by yourself," I frantically asked my brave little seven year old trooper. His eyes widened real big, lifting his head back and nodding up and down. "Yes mommy, I can do it, I know where it is," he insisted, eager to please and prove himself to me.

"Run straight to grandma's house as fast as you can. When you get there, go to the garage and tell papa that mommy's mobile home is on fire. Tell him to bring pliers and shovels right away. Do you understand me, Jimmy? Don't forget what I told you, and don't forget to tell him we need pliers. I have to have pliers to turn the water on. Go now, and run as fast as you can, and Jimmy, remember to watch for cars," I shouted, turning his little shoulders to shove him off in the right direction.

"Okay mommy, I'll hurry," he said, bravely running off to save the day. I watched as he sprinted across the desert floor, his short little legs stretched to their limits in every stride and effort toward the next step as he ran for papa's help.

"Granny, watch Jeffrey," I ordered, running back home. I ran to the back yard and saw that the fence was now completely engulfed in flames. The hot red and yellow flames beat against the walls of my mobile home spitting hot embers at me. We were going to lose our home, any second now. I ran around the yard desperately searching for the pliers. I frantically begged God, "Please help me to find the pliers!"

Not knowing what to do next, I ran outside whispering, "Please God, don't burn down our home and take everything from us because of what I did. I won't have an abortion, I promise! I'll do whatever you say. I'm sorry, I'm sorry, I'm so sorry, please God!" As the words tumbled from my lips, I looked down the middle of the road to see an unfamiliar stranger strolling toward me, very slowly. For a brief moment, he was all I could see. I felt drawn to him for some unexplainable reason and I knew I had to run to him for help. He walked with a casual, methodical stride, piercing me with his eyes with every measured step he took toward me.

Not recognizing the stranger from anywhere in our small community, I quickly ran toward him. "Sir, do you have a pair of pliers? I need pliers to turn my water on before my trailer burns down," I pleaded. I stood watching him with a fearful regret for yelling at God in such a disrespectful, and rebellious manner.

The stranger, never speaking a word, nodded yes and turned back to get pliers. "Please hurry before my trailer burns down," I cried after him, alarmed.

I ran back into my yard to wait for the stranger's return, while I continued to search for the missing pliers. I looked under the trailer, kicking sand around in desperate frustration. They were nowhere to be found. The stranger hadn't returned and I ran back to the street to search for him. I stopped in the road and saw him walking toward me. I watched as he continued to walk in the slow, casual, measured step that he did when I first spotted him. "Why isn't he running? Can't he see my mobile home is about to burn down?" I thought. With an overpowering panic for the pliers, I ran to the stranger, yelling "Thank you," as I snatched the pliers from his hand.

I ran to the spigot. My heart pounded against my chest so hard, it felt as though a two hundred pound man was center punching me in the middle of my chest. My hands trembled fiercely as I twisted the pliers to turn the water on. I grabbed the hose and ran for the back yard, spraying the water on the burning fence, in an attempt to drown the fire. The wind picked up, blowing the flames toward me, stopping me from getting close enough to spray water on to the fire. The heat from the flames was singing the hair on my flesh, driving me back, until I could no longer get close enough with the hose to douse the fire. I watched as the flames prepared to engulf my home any second and cried out, "Please God, help me!" I pressed harder and deeper into the end of the hose, with my thumb, trying to make the water reach further. I cried out once more, "Please God, don't take everything we have from us now. I promise, I will not have an abortion!"

I heard a strong, authoritative voice commanding obedience, say to me, "Give that to me," and grabbed the hose from my hand. His face wore the look of authority and confidence, as one in complete control of the circumstances. For a brief second, as our eyes met, I thought I could see his disappointment in me. I wondered if maybe it was because I couldn't get close enough to the fire to put it out, or did he know? "Did he know about the fit I'd just had with God? How could he know? Did he over hear me screaming at God? He couldn't have over heard me." I thought quietly. Curious about this man, and very grateful, I continued to watch as he stepped forward, up to the flames, dousing them with the hose.

I gazed at him in amazement as he stepped nearly into the flames, spraying the fire with water. I couldn't believe the flames weren't burning him. Suddenly aware of someone stepping in behind me, I turned to see my step father come in with three or four men, all with shovels throwing dirt on the fire in an attempt to suffocate it. One neighbor had grabbed his hose, connected it to the spigot on the empty lot east of me. Everyone compassionately and diligently worked to save my home, helping to fight the flames of destruction.

Before I knew it, the flames were out. I stood in awe of how many people had come to rescue my home. I walked over to the water spigot and turned the water off. I carried the stranger's pliers in my hand so I could return it. I had seen trailers burn to the ground in our little town of Cabazon, but I had never seen so many others come to the rescue as I had seen today. Truly God's hand was over my undeserving life this day. My thoughts turned toward Granny, who watched my children across the street. Not long ago, her own mobile home had burned to the ground. She lost everything. In the terrifying experience of today's events, I had a new compassion for her.

I turned to see everyone who had come to my aid, helping me to put the fire out. We were every one of us, covered with sweat and dirt, and some of us were wet from the spray of the hose. We were all feeling excited in our triumph over the fire. I was exhausted from the physical, and emotional ordeal of this terrifying experience. I walked over to thank each person, individually, for their assistance. I couldn't have done it alone. I joined my step father, who stood on the walkway, leading to the porch. He asked how it happened. I said I had no idea, but deep down inside, I knew all along it was God. I just didn't see how I could explain this to anyone. The boys were in the house with me. We had just returned home a few minutes before the fire started. I told him about the stranger who had brought me the pliers.

"Where is he now?" he asked.

I don't know," I replied. I felt a peace fall over me such as I had never felt before and I could feel the presence of God. I searched the yard for the stranger, realizing I had not yet thanked him. I saw him standing at the front gate, his eyes piercing me once again. I was very grateful to the stranger for everything he did to help me. His stare made me feel a need to explain, or apologize, or something. I pointed him out to my step-father, and said, "I need to go over there to thank him and return his pliers."

"I'll go with you," my step father said. "Who is he? I've never seen him before. I want to meet him," he muttered curiously as he followed me to the gate. I found it very odd that my step father didn't know the man, considering he has known every person in Cabazon for as long as I can remember. We used to visit his best friend when there were no more than half a dozen homes in Cabazon. Between them, they knew everyone then, and everyone since.

I felt intimidated by the stranger's piercing eyes. I had the feeling he was someone important, someone of great authority. There was just something so different about him. I sheepishly approached him, thanking him and reached out my hand with the pliers. "Thank you so much for helping me. You don't know how much I appreciate it. I don't think I could have done it by myself," I said, feeling very humbled.

The stranger reached out and gently removed the pliers from my hand. His voice thundered with a reprimanding tone as he said with a stern, demanding voice, "Don't you thank me young lady. You know who it is you are to thank for this!"

The stranger never broke his gaze from mine. I felt his eyes penetrate, cutting through to the quickening of my very soul. Suddenly, I was fearful and didn't understand why. My mouth fell open and my lips were moving, but no sound came from throat. The fear of the Lord had fallen upon me. I could not break my eyes away from the penetration of his glare. I stepped back away from him.

My step father stepped toward the stranger out of curiosity. He said to the stranger, "I don't know you from around here. What's your name?"

The stranger moved his gaze from my eyes to my step father. With great kindness and compassion he said aloud, "You don't need to know my name. My name doesn't matter here!" He turned his face back toward mine, stared directly into my eyes and said again, "You know to whom you are to go to give your thanks!"

My step father looked toward the ground, concentrating, trying to recall if he had ever seen this man before. He spoke up once more and said, "Can I ask where you live? Do you live around here?"

The stranger turned toward the southwest. He appeared to be pointing across the street, two doors down from Granny's home. "Over there," he told us.

We turned to look in the direction his finger was pointing. The stranger turned and gazed into my eyes once more, leaving me speechless and turned to walk away.

I turned back to my step father and said, "That man does not live in that house." He agreed with me. We knew our neighbors and he was not one of them. "Maybe we misunderstood, and he is visiting someone there," I said.

We returned to my yard to collect the shovels and return to the truck. Meanwhile, I walked back out to the street to look for the stranger again. He was nowhere in sight. I walked across to thank Granny for all her help and returned home with the boys.

Just then, the fire trucks pulled up and the firemen entered my yard. They questioned me and checked to be sure the fire was completely out. They said the fire was started by the visiting grandchildren of the woman who lived behind me. They were playing with matches next to the fence and things got out of control. The fireman said it was definitely a miracle. He had never seen a trailer survive a fire like this one. They complimented us on a job well done and returned to their trucks.

Michael returned home just in time to see the fire trucks and ran through the front gate yelling, "What happened? Is everyone okay? Judith, where are the kids? Are they okay?" He panicked and turned to take a stance, ready to lunge and protect as he looked around, absorbing the sights surrounding him.

A Fireman approached Michael, reassuring him that everything was okay. He explained what had happened, shook Michael's hand, and joined the others in the truck. Jimmy and Jeffrey excitedly ran after the truck, waving good bye to the firemen as they drove away.

Michael and I took the boys and returned indoors. Before I could even sit down, Michael asked, "Judith, did you go to the clinic? Did you have the abortion? I know it's a girl, Judith!" Michael asked, upset about the abortion.

"Michael, you won't believe what happened. I can hardly believe it myself and I was there! It's just too weird," I exclaimed, totally exhausted. I went on to tell Michael about Sylvia's car not starting.

He smiled and said, "I told you God wants us to have this baby! I don't know how I know, but it's a girl! I am certain, it's a girl!"

"Be quiet and let me finish. You won't believe this." I continued to give him the details of the day's events, right down to my defiance against God. "I couldn't believe God didn't strike me dead," I confessed. I told him about the stranger and pointed out the window to the house across the street, I said, "He said he lives over there, but I know he doesn't live across the street, Michael. Not unless he is an Angel living there."

Michael got up to see which mobile home I was pointing to and said, "Nobody like that lives over there, Judith. Maybe you misunderstood?" He gazed at me questionably?

"I didn't misunderstand anything. You can ask my step father, George. He knows everybody in this town and he doesn't know him, and furthermore, nobody here today has ever seen that man before.

Michael, I can't explain it, but I think this man is not a man at all, but an angel sent by God. There was something about his piercing, convicting eyes and the way he spoke. He spoke with great authority and I felt as though I was being warned by him. I felt an awe and a fearful, healthy respect every time he spoke," I attempted to explain. I really do believe he is an angel sent by God. I don't get it. I was cursing and threatening God up one side and down the other today. I don't know why He didn't completely wipe out everything, including me. I deserve His wrath, but instead, he saved me.

We agreed that from that moment on, we would spy on the neighbors and find out who this stranger is.

"Well, one thing hasn't changed, I still don't want another kid, but I promised God that if he saved our home, I would not abort and I won't. I just can't reconcile myself to having another child. I am hopelessly unhappy and afraid. I don't know what I am going to do yet, but I'll figure it out," I confided in my exhaustion. "I guess there is always a chance I could still miscarry and if not, there is always adoption. Maybe God intends on another family adopting it," I said.

Completely exhausted, I told him I had to lay down as I fell across the sofa. Michael ordered me to lay there and rest while he made dinner for us.

We sat down to eat, and Jimmy and Jeffrey were still excited about seeing the firemen. They continued to share every minutia of the day's events over dinner. Jimmy, so proudly detailed how he did just what mommy told him. "I ran all the way to grandma's house really fast, and I only stopped to look for cars. I remembered exactly how to get there, too," Jimmy exclaimed! "I helped papa put shovels in the truck and watched my brother so he wouldn't get hurt. I was a good boy today," Jimmy boasted proudly.

With a sudden burst of energy, Jeffrey piped, "Jesus helped mommy too, daddy," he sputtered with a mouth full of food.

"All the glory belongs to Jesus! He protects us, and you were both hero's today. I am so proud of both of you," Michael smiled at the boys.

We sent the boys to bathe after dinner and retired to the living room to watch TBN on television. I couldn't stop thinking about the day's events, in particularly, the stranger. Why didn't our trailer catch fire? I watched the flames beat against the side of the trailer over, and over. The entire day was such a mystery. There was no other explanation, it was definitely God's handiwork.

Over the next few days, the fire became the buzz of the week in Cabazon. Everybody was talking about it. Periodically, friends and locals asked about the fire and how it happened. We would explain and ask each one about the stranger. The funny thing is, nobody, had any idea who he was. We continued to spy on the house across the street. We never did see anyone that even remotely resembled the stranger go in, or out of that house.

Weeks passed, and I prayerfully begged God for a miscarriage. The boys played in their room as I sat alone in the quiet, with my thoughts. I dwelled in my own self-pity and fear, angry at God for forcing me to have another child. I fought to force my anger back down, asking Jesus to forgive me. I was afraid to say how I really felt out loud again, for fear of God striking me dead where I stood and sending me to hell. After all, God was always looking for a reason to send to me to hell. God knows, I have given Him enough reasons to do it. It didn't matter anymore, I knew Jesus understood and would help me. He loved and understood me and didn't want me to go to hell. He even died on the cross so I wouldn't have to go to hell.

I suddenly remembered my mother telling me when I was a young girl about some home remedies that would help me to self-induce a miscarriage. She had said that if I take a bunch of aspirin and drank a coke very quickly, it would bring on a miscarriage, or I could drink castor oil and it would cause a miscarriage as well. I knew there was no castor oil in the kitchen, but I found the bottle of aspirin. I took out ten aspirin and opened a coke. I swallowed the aspirin and quickly guzzled the coke and I waited.

The hours passed, and nothing. Nothing at all, not even the hope that it would happen. I was so overwhelmed with the fear of having another child, I was desperate to try anything to stop this pregnancy from happening. I decided to help the aspirin and coke out by running hard and fast around the double lot that our mobile home sat on. I continued to run until I was out of breath and couldn't run anymore. I waited for any sign of blood or cramps, and nothing. It seemed the only thing I had accomplished was physical exertion, and for naught. I managed to close the doors of my mind's misery and focus on the chores that needed to be done.

Michael returned from work and shared the new recipes he had created, announcing his employer was so impressed with his culinary arts that they had given Michael a fifty cent an hour increase in wage. We cheered for him and agreed to have a special, celebratory dinner in his honor. Michael perked up and suggested we go to town to purchase items for his to recreate his newest version of, "Beef Stroganoff."

"Yeah, yeah, yeah," Jimmy sang out, jumping up and down in excitement and grabbing Michael's hands. Jeffrey jumped right in, mimicking his brother, and the three of them danced.

We entered the grocery store, searching every aisle for the necessary items. Suddenly Michael seemed detached from our little celebration and I asked, "What's wrong?"

Michael was unable to hold eye contact with me. He stood with one hand on the cart, the other in his pocket, and turned his head to look at items on a shelf. He hesitated and said, "Well, this is such a special occasion, I want to buy a six pack of beer to celebrate my raise."

Feeling overwhelmed with the fear of his drinking again, I felt the need to get control of the situation. "What are you thinking, Michael? You are an alcoholic. You can never drink again. You know you won't be able to stop at a six pack," I insisted. "You promised you would never drink again, Michael. Why are you doing this?" My mood had suddenly turned very hostile.

"Never mind," he retorted. I can go without it. I just thought a couple of beer would taste good and got a little too excited about our celebration. I'm sorry. Let's just go home now," he voiced somberly. This confirmed to me, exactly why we shouldn't have another child. The thought of three children and a practicing alcoholic husband terrified me. Having another child now, for me, would be like having four children as a single mother, with the oldest child running amuck and out of control.

After unloading the groceries, Michael made dinner, and took great satisfaction in his wonderful new version of

Beef Stroganoff. We sat down at the table, prayed, and praised Michael for a job well done. Jimmy and Jeffrey proclaimed it was the best dinner they ever had, stopping to rub their tummies and exclaiming, "Yummmmmy," after every bite.

Later that evening we sat down to share our thoughts. "Michael, do you feel like drinking again? What's going on with you? Do you need an A.A. meeting?" I asked suggestively.

"Yeah, I probably do need a meeting. I will go to the ten o'clock meeting in the morning," he said stretching his neck to lean his head on the back of the sofa in an attempt to escape the evening, remaining somber and withdrawn.

Michael was working part time and attending several A.A. meetings a week. I had become uneasy when he was out of my sight. I became suspicious of his whereabouts when he said he was attending meetings. My gut instinct was taking over and the red warning lights were flashing in my mind, filling my heart with doubt and confusion. We retired to our bed where I gently arranged my foot across his leg, convincing myself that if he moved or got up, I would awaken and stop him from drinking.

The bright, rich morning rays of the sun penetrated through the gaps of the floral print curtains, resting across my face as I felt its warmth settling upon my cheeks. My foot still laid across Michael's leg causing me to recall our conversation from the night before. I lived in an all-consuming fear of Michael's abandonment, binge drinking, thievery, and the other temporary female companions he visited on occasion. I stopped trusting him a long time ago and had forgotten how to trust anyone. I had come to view my little world with a cynical disdain for men, and relationships. I was determined to stop Michael from destroying our lives with his ghastly, overpowering addictions.

With all trust gone, so was the niceties in the demands I placed on him. Since our heart to heart talks failed, I used threats to try and stop Michael. I would threaten to end our relationship and throw him out, never to return again. I threatened to never let him see our children again. I even threatened him with a baseball bat and yes, even his life. It didn't seem to matter what I threatened him with, he jeered at my threats and continued to fall prey to his addictions in short periodicals.

I watched Michael, who slept so peacefully beside me and my heart cried. I snuggled up against him, closing my eyes and envisioned myself merging my body into his and becoming one with him. I wondered if he truly knew just how much I really, really loved him. If I could just get inside of him, he would know. Then we would become one and nobody, or nothing could separate us, not even that bottle of booze.

I pressed into Michael, wondering if he knew that every time I attacked him, I was really attacking the booze and his addictions, and not him. I just didn't know any other way and never meant to hurt him. I loved him so much, it hurt. Sometimes, I wanted him to know the pain he inflicted on me and our children. I keep forgiving him, but he keeps on doing the same things, again and again. "You would think he would of learned by now, shoot, you would think I would of learned by now," and people wonder why I am so angry. If they only knew, or understood what I've lived with these past seven years.

I heard the pitter patter of little feet running the length of the trailer, coming toward my room. I gently pulled away from Michael and quickly darted into the living room to greet the morning with Jimmy and Jeffrey.

"Shhhh, don't wake up dad. He's still sleeping," I cautioned the boys. I started our morning routine and Michael arose, planting himself on the sofa as I handed him a fresh cup of coffee. "Are you still going to a meeting?" I asked him.

"That is why I got up," he retorted, He dressed and left for the morning A.A. meeting. I sat on the sofa wondering if he would return home today, or leave on another bender.

I sent the boys off to their room to play for a while and stood on the front porch alone with my fears and thoughts. I looked at the railroad ties stacked against the three foot high, wooden slab that served as our porch. I was desperate and wondered if throwing myself down the sharp steps, would cause me to miscarry.

I walked back to the wall, took a deep breath and made a short run, tossing myself from the top of the steps, tumbling downward. I had scraped my arm in the fall and other than that, I felt fine. I walked to the top of the steps and repeated the same maneuver, but threw myself harder this time, landing on my side. I stood up and remained motionless, waiting. "Man alive, this is a strong pregnancy and it is really hanging on," I thought. "I can't have another baby, please God, don't make me have another one. I just can't do this," I cried out with waves of immense anger rushing over me like a tidal wave.

I sat down on the sofa and waited. I waited for Michael to return. I waited to see if I would miscarry. I waited for Michael to quit drinking. I waited for lunch to feed the boys. It seemed, I was always waiting for something, or someone. "I am so tired of waiting, of always waiting," I thought quietly.

I sent the boys back outside after lunch, rubbing my scraped, painful elbow and worried about Michael. I prayed, "Please God, bring him home."

That afternoon, Michael staggered through the door reeking of whiskey with his red, cloudy eyes, unfocused.

"Why? Why did you do this? You said you were going to a meeting. I knew you were lying. You promised to stay sober," I screamed vehemently.

He leaned, cocking his head back, as he did whenever he was confronted. I wasn't drinking! I don't know what you're talking about and you're always accusing me. I'm sick of it," he slurred, hitting my chest to knock me away from him.

"Michael, I can smell the whiskey! You liar! Don't tell me someone in A.A. was drinking whiskey and spilled it on you. You didn't go to a meeting. You went across the street to the bar. Liar! How can I trust you, or believe anything you say ever again! You are a lousy, sloppy, disgusting drunk with a split tongue! The devil's tongue. Sometimes, I think you are Satan himself and I hate your guts," I reviled against him, throwing my bible across the room.

"I'm sorry, Judy! I'm sorry," he sputtered in his drunken drawl, rocking back and forth, attempting to maintain his balance. I've been going to the bar instead of meetings for a couple of weeks now," he confessed.

"Oh my God! How could I have not known until now? THE MONEY! Where did he get the money?" I thought for a moment.

"The rent money? Where is it, Michael? Where is our money? You better not have spent it," I yelled from the burning, hollowed depths of my belly! "Give it to me," I demanded!

He pursed his lips, turning his glazed eyes toward me in a slumbered gaze, and said, "I spent it."

"All of it? Did you spend all of it? What about groceries, food for the kids? What about our rent, Michael? How will we pay rent?" I questioned furiously.

"I'll figure something out, Judy. Don't worry about it. I'll find side jobs and put the money back. I promise you," he said.

"Oh God, can't you see why we can't have this baby? I can see the headlines now," I sarcastically stated. "BABY DIES OF STARVATION WHILE FATHER SITS IN DRUNKEN STUPOR, news at Eleven!" I continued to rant, "I threw myself down the steps today, Michael, trying to create a miscarriage. You better pray we don't have another kid. The last thing we need is to bring another kid into this mess," I screamed.

"What? Why would you do that? You could have hurt yourself," his words slurred barely audible.

"Look at you, and you have to ask me that?" I continued the verbal assaults and walked outside, enraged.

"I have a doctor's appointment in the morning and will be taking the car. I'm going to lay down, leave me alone," I shouted after walking back inside.

I sat in the doctor's office waiting for my name to be called, feeling impatient and nauseous. The nurse called my name, and performed the usual tasks.

I lay back on the examining table as Dr. Stanheiser pushed and prodded my belly. "Everything looks good. I will be leaving for a vacation tomorrow and will be gone for six weeks. If you have any problems while I am gone, don't hesitate to go to the emergency room. It looks like everything is going really well and I don't expect any problems. The front desk will give you the first available appointment after I return," she informed me. Looking over my chart again, she said, "Yes, you are five months along now. Go home and rest," she said walking out the door.

I returned home, feeling nauseous and dizzy. The boys ran to me, grabbed my legs and nearly knocked me to the floor.

"Hey boys, you're going to hurt mommy. Get off her like that," Michael warned. "What did the doc say?"

Everything is fine. She's going on vacation for six weeks, so I won't see her for a while. I'm feeling a little dizzy and nauseous with cramps. I don't remember feeling this way, this late in the pregnancy before. I'm going to go lay down.

Michael took the boys to the park and I wondered how much longer they would be gone. I felt weak and had no energy. I drank a cola, hoping the sugar help me.

Weeks passed and I wasn't feeling any better. In fact, I felt worse. I paid a visit to my mother, to ask her what she thought might be wrong with me.

Without ever looking up, my mother said, "I'd know those footsteps anywhere, hello Judith! Make yourself a cup of tea and join me."

I listened to her tales of the "Wheel Inn," truck stop where she was employed. Mom had six children. If anyone would know what was wrong with me, she would.

I shared my symptoms with her and she was unable to come to any conclusions. "I guess I'll have to wait for Dr. Stanheiser to return," I said, and returned home.

Michael received a paycheck and we were sorely in need of groceries. What I didn't tell my mother was, I didn't feel strong enough to go to the store alone anymore.

We all piled in the car and headed for the grocery store in town. Once inside, I held on to the cart tightly, allowing the cool air to blow over me. I felt very overheated from the drive. It had turned very warm outside and we didn't have air conditioning in that old Mercury. Suddenly, I became very dizzy. The room began to spin, my head was pounding and I felt nauseous again. I held on to the cart, feeling incredibly weak and forced myself to continue walking up and down the aisles with Michael and the boys, as I attempted to hide my symptoms.

Chapter 4
NEAR DEATH

The odor of barbeque sauce mingled with varying spices, filling the air. The different scents of various pre-cooked meats on the end cap of the aisle started to weigh heavily on my senses. Jimmy, who was always eager to please, searched for items on our grocery list with Michael, unaware of my struggle for consciousness.

Jeffrey sat in the front of the grocery cart, vying for my attention with his beautifully dimpled smile and twinkling eyes. He teased me with his smile, and I attempted to smile back at him. Suddenly, something was very wrong. I had never felt like this before. "Am I going to die? Am I finally losing the baby? Oh God, what is happening to me?" I fearfully cried from the deepest recesses of my mind.

I bent over to the bottom shelf, pushing the canned goods to the floor. "I need a place to sit down," I barely whispered. My head fell back, as my body reeled in an unbalanced motion, and I reached one hand out for Michael who stood a distance from me. I drew in a long, deep, slow breath while groveling for the side of the cart with my other hand. I felt as if I were battling for my life. I had to win this battle and I struggled for control over my body.

I bent over to sit down on the empty shelf, grabbing the side of the cart to guide me. I heard a woman's voice speak, "Is she alright?" Her voice sounded out in my head, as if it were reverberating out of a small chamber, echoing through my mind. I felt a heaviness come over me, and darkness blanketed my eyes. I felt myself slowly, slipping away. I could no longer hold on, slumping over the floor as the lower shelf caught the upper part of my body. I continued to struggle with this unknown entity that overtook my senses, as I slipped into the vast darkness of fear.

Michael was holding my head in his hand, and with his other hand, he patted my cheeks, while calling my name aloud. I heard Jimmy and Jeffrey crying, as I slowly returned to full consciousness. I became more aware of my surroundings as I listened to Michael tell the boys, "Mommy is okay!" I scurried to my feet in embarrassment, announcing I was fine. Still weak, I asked Michael for a cold soda. He raced off to find one for me when I realized my entire body was shaking and I clung desperately to the cart for balance. I drank the cold soda quickly, allowing the sugar to lift me. I felt a little stronger when I noticed Jimmy's hand held tightly to my wrist, guarding me with his protective little hands. I looked into his beautiful, deep set, blue eyes and saw the fearful concern for his mommy. I reassured him that I was okay and drew both the boys in close to me, holding them tightly against my side.

By the time we had returned home, the onset of dizziness had returned. It seemed I was either dizzy or suffering vertigo, more than not. I began to experience leg cramps, heavy breathing, blurred vision and severe headaches all the time, not to mention the nausea. I had trouble lifting myself to my own my feet, on along walking anywhere.

I went into the kitchen to empty the grocery bags. I sorted the items and handed them off to the boys to put away. Michael had turned on television to watch sports. We purchased our ground beef in bulk, often as much as 30 lbs. at a time. When we had less money, we purchased 15 lbs. This was a 15 lb. shopping trip. I would divide the ground beef into one lb. packages for freezing and we would laugh at the idea of writing a book titled, "1,001 Ways to Prepare Ground Beef."

I divided the ground beef into piles on the table and stood to reach for the freezer wrap, when my battle for consciousness began, once again. I was sure I was departing from my body and going to die this time.

I turned around in an attempt to make it back to my chair when I slid down the cupboard, to the floor. I heard Jimmy scream, "DADDY!" Jumping up and down, he cried out, "Daddy, mommy fell on the floor and I think she's hurt." Never fully reaching unconsciousness, I felt a slight awareness of the voices and noises surrounding me but was too weak to hold myself up.

Michael ran into the kitchen and kneeled in front of me to ask, "Are you okay? What happened, Judith? I think you need to call your doctor," he said, concerned.

"I'm okay, I'm just pregnant," I light heartedly remarked. "Will you help me to the sofa?"

He lifted me from the floor and carried me to the sofa, where he laid me. I asked for another cold soda. "You shouldn't be drinking so many of those," he said.

"Whenever I drink a soda, I feel better. The sugar rush helps me to get moving and makes me feel more energized again," I explained.

I think these are just pregnancy symptoms for which I don't have any pregnancy solutions right now," I said jokingly with a weak voice. I giggled at myself, attempting to relieve his concerns with humor.

"Every pregnancy is different, and this pregnancy has been nothing like my other pregnancies. It will get better soon," I assured him, trying to hide my own concern. I returned to the kitchen to finish packaging the ground beef.

I spent most days sitting comfortably in my rocker, unable to move around because of the dizziness and varying symptoms I had been experiencing. When I wasn't in my rocker, I was laying on the sofa, begging someone to bring me a soda to re-energize me.

On several occasions, Michael had returned home reeking of alcohol. I knew he was drinking, but I was too weak to fight with him. I would mention smelling the alcohol and he would fervently deny drinking. I felt he was taking advantage of my weakened condition and at the same time, I was grateful he came home, instead of taking off on another bender.

There were only two weeks until Dr. Stanheiser returned and I thought I would feel better as the pregnancy progressed. So much for what I thought! I was feeling much worse. The multiple symptoms in my body increased, while my energy levels and strength continually decreased. I didn't trust myself to drive a car because the dizziness and vertigo were relentlessly unending. Every time I drank a soda, I felt better, but shortly thereafter, the symptoms would return again with a vengeance. It was time to reveal the truth to Michael. I was frightened and began to ponder thoughts of cancer, or some unknown disease that was continually assaulting my body. I was convinced that God was going to slay me, and make me suffer in the process for being disrespectful, and rebellious toward Him.

Michael returned from work, his face red from the heat. He sat shirtless in front of the fan, attempting to cool down and relax. I gazed at him, wondering what he would do if something were to happen to me. Would he abandon the boys the same way he repeatedly abandoned me whenever he had an urge for another bender?

I knew Michael would never be able to care for our sons alone. I opened a conversation with him, explaining the symptoms I was experiencing. I confided that I had been feeling much worse lately, and was developing more symptoms than "Carter had liver pills," if that were possible.

I told him that I was confused. I was afraid there was nothing wrong with me, and I was acting like a hypochondriac. In contradiction, I told him I was afraid there was something really wrong with me, or the baby, and that, "something," would be very serious.

"I have never experienced anything like this, and I don't know what to relate it to. I am taking my vitamins, and eating right, but there is something..... Something just doesn't feel right. I guess I will have to trust God, and wait until Dr. Stanheiser returns, to find out what is wrong, if anything," I openly confided.

"With every bout for consciousness, I feel as though I am departing from my own body, barely holding on. I have passed out before, but this is very different. I literally feel as if I am passing from my body," I continued. "It's really weird and I can't exactly explain it, because I don't understand it myself," I told him. "The more I think about it, the more afraid I become. What if I have developed cancer or some other wretched disease? I have never known anyone with these symptoms before, so, I have nothing, or nobody to correlate it to. I can't drive anymore, and I can barely walk on my own," I complained. We prayed for healing and deliverance of whatever had attached itself to me. We asked the Lord for strength, and to uphold me until Dr. Stanheiser returned.

"Judith, tomorrow is our Friday morning prayer meeting at church. I think we should both go and ask Pastor Browning to pray over you," Michael suggested, greatly concerned.

I didn't want to tell the church about my dilemma. They were always trying to hug me or touch me, and I was always pushing them away. I didn't like to be touched or hung on by anyone, not even my own children. Michael pressured me until I gave in and agreed to his appeal.

"I'll go for you. Are you happy now? I smirked, agreeing to his request and appreciative of his concern.

The following morning, Michael drove us to the little white church that sat at the end of the road, beside the freeway. He walked me through the doors of the church with his arm around my waist to support me, and his other hand over my belly, to balance me. Members of our church greeted us, still attempting to hug me. I had learned how to put up my hand, and avert my eyes, as if to say "Stop!" They would recognize the hand signal, smile and politely shake my hand.

When Pastor Browning asked for prayer requests, Michael told the congregated prayer warriors attending that morning about my dilemma. He described my battle for consciousness, the feeling that something was very wrong and that my doctor would not be returning from vacation for a couple of weeks, yet.

Sister Mary Nell, Pastor Browning's wife, along with the other prayer warriors approached, encircling me as they began to pray against the menacing symptoms that hindered me. Afterwards, Mary Nell felt an urgency to continue to pray for me. They agreed to do just that, until my doctor returned and routinely checked in on me by phone.

With each passing day, the symptoms didn't seem to get any better, but at least they weren't getting any worse. Every morning, someone from church called on our newly installed telephone to pray with me. Michael felt, our money was best spent on a telephone, considering my condition. John and Joyce would come to our home several times a week to lay hands on, and pray over me. John was an elder in our church and Joyce was his wife with whom we had become very close friends. I became more resolved to the pregnancy, each time someone prayed over me.

The symptoms remained in strength, regardless of our prayers, yet the Lord gave me a peace about it. My concerned mother, called to check on me every day, several times a day.

There were many concerned friends, relatives and neighbors. Sylvia came by periodically to visit. She was not a Christian, and I used our time together to witness to her.

Michael continued to drink, blaming it on his fear and the pressure of my illness. He confessed, he was afraid something was going to happen to me. He promised once again, to return to A.A. and stay sober.

Morning's light peeked in as I awoke to Jimmy and Jeffrey, each laying on either side of me. Jeffrey, propped on his elbows with his chin resting on his hands, smiled at me. Jimmy lay on the other side, playing with my hair. "I love you, mommy," Jeffrey whispered as he pressed his dimpled cheek into my shoulder. "I love you too, Mommy," Jimmy said, raising up to his knees, grabbing my hand to play with my fingers. "Can you get up now, mommy?" Jimmy asked.

"I love you too," I replied, reaching over to pull my sons into my bosom. We laid together, cuddling for a moment before I pulled them away to look at their faces. I asked, "How would you like to have a little sister or brother soon? You guys know, there is a baby in my tummy, right?"

Jeffrey excitedly shook his head and Jimmy silently stared at me, with a look of uncertainty. I provoked the boys into a discussion about their new little brother, or sister. It was obvious to me that God was going to make me have this baby, and I wanted to know how the boys felt about it.

"Daddy thinks the baby is a girl, and I think it is a boy. Do you think it's a little brother, or a little sister?" They looked at me as if they were trying to find a missing puzzle piece.

"Okay, which one do you want? Do you want a little brother, or a little sister?" Jeffrey shrugged his shoulders and smiled as though it didn't matter to him, one way or the other. "I want a baby," Jeffrey said, bobbing his head up and down in excitement.

Jimmy, with a staid look on his face, said, "If I have to have a baby, I want a brother. If you give me a little sister, I'll hate her and I will never like her," he forcefully stated. All girls do is pull hair. I don't care, I will never like her. I will hit her and be mean to her," Jimmy snapped.

"Don't worry, Jimmy! If it's a girl, I won't let her pull your beautiful, curly, blonde locks, but I think it is a boy. No matter, you will soon have a little sister or brother.

The baby started kicking my belly rambunctiously. "Here," I said, grabbing their hands and placing them on my belly. "Do you feel that? It's the baby kicking me." Jeffrey, excitedly leapt to his knees, took a deep breath and yelled, "Oh, Jesus loves my baby," pointing toward heaven with his other hand. Jimmy withdrew his hand and ran to the living room, leaving Jeffrey to take my hand, and guardedly walk me to my rocker.

"Do you want me to make you some tea, mommy?" Jimmy asked, taking on the role of the little man who would take care of, and protect his mommy. "No," I answered. "You are too young to be turning the stove on, young man," I said reproving him while pulling him in to me for a hug. "I love you so much," I growled playfully, squeezing him tightly.

"I love you most," Jeffrey blurted out with a giggle.

"I love you mostest," Jimmy charged loudly.

"No way, I love you the mostest, and the bestest, and the biggest, all the way to eternity and back, and you can't love me more than that," I firmly established, and we gigged playfully together.

There was a knock at the door. Sylvia was visiting several times a week, helping to watch me and the boys while Michael worked. I continued to witness to her during our visits, hoping she would see how badly we all needed Jesus in our lives.

Before long, Michael returned home, Sylvia left, and John and Joyce paid a visit to fellowship, and pray over me. I informed everyone that I had called Dr. Stanheiser's office and she would return this coming Tuesday. I was told she was very busy, just returning and all, but they moved me to her first available appointment time. I was going in on Tuesday morning to see her. I thanked John and Joyce for all their love, prayers and concern. They told us before leaving that they would be returning on Saturday to pray for me again.

Every so often, Michael would find a reason to leave without the kids, and return smelling like alcohol. He had been unsuccessful with attaining sobriety, "but at least he was trying," I thought to myself. My biggest fear right now, was that he would leave for a pack of cigarettes and not return, leaving me alone to fend for myself.

John and Joyce unexpectedly returned on Tuesday morning to pray for me before seeing Dr. Stanheiser. I knew it was the perpetual prayers that was holding me up. I was anxious about seeing the doctor. I couldn't wait on one hand, and scared to death she was going to tell me I was dying on the other hand. I was so very tired of the weakness, and feeling sick all the time. In my nervousness, I snapped at anyone who came near me that morning.

Michael checked me in at the window after guiding me into a chair in the waiting area. I waited for nearly an hour before my name was called.

Michael stood me up and walked me to the nurse. She took my arm and said, "I'll take her from here." I was escorted down the long corridor, to an examining room, only stopping long enough to have me stand on a scale. "Do you feel able to do this?" she asked.

"Yes, I think I can do it, if you will take my purse for me," I muttered weakly.

She measured me at 5'6" and weighed me at 108 pounds. Once we were in the examining room, she asked about the symptoms I was experiencing. I listed a few, not revealing everything, for fear she would think that I was a hypochondriac.

"Do you need help undressing, or will you be okay on your own?" The nurse inquired.

"I'll be okay," I replied, my entire body visibly shaking from weakness. I removed my clothing and laid on the examining table, covering myself with the paper sheet. My head was throbbing. I was cold and miserable, feeling confused and slightly disoriented as I waited for the doctor.

The door swung open as Dr. Stanheiser greeted me with a cheery, yet concerned, "Hello Judith, I see you're having some problems. Tell me, what's going on?"

"It seems like everything is wrong," I replied.

Dr. Stanheiser questioned me about the symptoms I had reported to the nurse. She asked if I had experienced any other symptoms. She named a few, such as; trembling, anxiety, palpitations, cold or clammy, numbness, pins and needles, as if my limbs had fallen asleep.

"Yes, to all of those," I answered. "Wow! How did you know?" I questioned in amazement.

She continued, "What about leg cramps, abdominal discomfort, nausea, vomiting, dizziness, vertigo, headaches, lethargy, mood swings, confusion, delirium, fatigue, or blurred vision," she called out each symptom as she marked them on my chart, when I responded yes to every one of them.

"What is wrong with me? Is it serious? How did you know I was having all those symptoms?" I queried. "I am so tired of feeling ill and in pain all the time," I remarked, relieved to find I wasn't a hypochondriac after all.

"It's my job to know these things," she smiled. "Now lean back and let's take a look at you and your baby," she ordered confidently.

Dr. Stanheiser finished my exam, left the room and returned a few minutes later with my blood and urine results. She questioned me about my diet. "What have you been eating and drinking, and how many times a day?" I listed everything, including how many soda's I drank a day.

She lowered her head while intently listening to me and reached for my chart, looking it over again. "Judith, it looks like you have Hypoglycemia," she said.

"hy, hy, hyper what?" I stuttered, curiously ignorant. "I have never heard that word before. What is it?"

"Hypoglycemia," she said again. It is low blood sugar, not to be confused with Hyperglycemia or Diabetes.

I know what diabetes is, I am very familiar with it. My step-father has Diabetes," I told her.

"Okay then, Hypoglycemia is the opposite of what Diabetes is. There is no medication for it and it is completely diet controlled," she informed me. "A normal blood sugar range is 80 to 130. Judith, I just checked your blood and urine results and your blood sugar reading is +4. To be perfectly frank and not to scare you, but I don't how you walked into my office. In fact, you are very lucky to be alive, on along conscious and surprisingly, walking," she said amazed. "How long have you been experiencing these symptoms?"

"About five weeks, it started right after you left for vacation," I answered her.

"Why didn't you go to the hospital? Judith, this is not good for you, or the baby. I am going to be blunt and brutally honest with you. This may have had some adverse effects on the baby. Have you felt the baby moving?" She asked with great concern.

"Yes, the baby has been kicking up a storm, flip flopping all the time, including hic-cups, which the baby generously shares with me every time. Why?"

"Judith, there is a risk that the child may be born with brain damage and the possibility of physical deformation. The baby has been deprived. As your blood glucose fluctuated, so did the baby's. It may have had a negative effect and the baby"......

"W...W... Wait," I interrupted. "Oh God!" Confused, I sat in disbelief as the shock from her words struck me. "I feel confused and I'm not sure I'm understanding you," my words trailed off in my confusion. "My husband is outside. Can you ask him to come in here and explain it to him? I'm not sure I'm completely getting it," I said with a disheartened emptiness. "Everyone in my church has been laying hands on me, calling me, and praying for me every day. I thought I was going to die," I blurted out, trying to change the subject back to me, in hopes of denying her diagnoses of the baby.

Dr. Stanheiser, smiled, patted my hand and said, "Prayer is probably the only reason you are still alive, Judith. I believe in prayer and I think you and your husband should continue to pray."

Michael entered the examining room, and my eyes welled up as I fought back the tears when I saw him. "No, no, no, I will not fall into this emotional sink hole. I will stay strong!"

Dr. Stanheiser rearranged my file in front of her and explained everything to Michael. She said we would have to wait until the child was born before discovering if there had been any injury, or adverse effect to the child. She said she would like to see my glucose levels remain between 90 and 110. She used Diabetes as a comparison, explaining that a blood glucose of 60 or below could result in insulin shock, and below 50 could result in coma or death. She recapped the seriousness of my condition and how very lucky I am.

"I am going to schedule you to see my dietician this Friday and I will schedule you for an ultra sound and a glucose test on Monday in my office. Michael, I want you to immediately fill your wife's tummy with a high protein meal immediately. Her blood sugar is out of control right now, endangering her and your child," she insisted. "Judith, no more sugar or soda pop for you! Understood?"

"I understand, but I don't know what I'm going to drink now. I hate water," I whimpered.

"You can drink juice but be careful," She warned. "Fruit contains natural sugar, nonetheless, it is sugar and will affect your glucose levels if you drink too much, or too fast. If there are any further complications, don't hesitate to go to ER. Do you have any other questions for me?"

"I don't think so," Michael said, thanking her for her patience with us.

I couldn't feel my legs under me as Michael walked me to the front desk, leading me by my arm.

We stopped for something quick and protein filled to take home to eat. I filled my belly as the doctor's words gnawed at me. The protein helped me to awaken my mind.

After arriving home, I walked to the refrigerator to pop open a soda. "I love soda pop and I'm not going to completely stop drinking them," I rebelliously announced.

Dodging Michael's reach, as his arm swept past me, I lifted the bottle to my mouth, stubbornly guzzling until I couldn't take the tickle in my nose any longer. All of a sudden, the room started moving, and I was dizzy again. "Okay, here you go. Maybe that wasn't such a good Idea," I said, handing the bottle over to Michael.

"That was a stupid thing to do," Michael angrily countered. "I'm going to make you something to eat," he said, handing me a slice of cheese to snack on. "Just sit there until I'm finished and no more sugar, Judith! I mean it," he demanded, his eyes fiercely scorning me.

"We need to talk about this," I called out to the kitchen, from my rocking chair.

"Wait until after lunch. We'll send the boys out to play and talk then," he adamantly called back. I was pleasantly surprised to see Michael taking charge since I was not accustomed to seeing him stand up to adversity. He usually left it up to me to handle all our problems as they arose.

After lunch, we discussed our plan to have a healthy baby. My heart was breaking and I wondered if I was being punished for attempting to abort, and not wanting another child. The doctor's words were reeling back and forth in my mind as I questioned everything all over again, but this time from a different perspective.

"I was having trouble accepting that I was going to have another baby to take care of, knowing that I already had two children and an alcoholic husband to care and provide for. How was I going to care and provide for a physically and mentally challenged baby, with two children and a drunk for a husband?" I thought to myself in bitter frustration.

Michael picked up his bible, and lifted his face as if to look toward God for an answer. "Judith, you need to accept that we are going to have this baby, and stop denying it. I don't care what anyone says. I know it's a girl, a daughter, our daughter. I know in my heart that she is okay. I don't believe what the doctor said, and I declare it to be a lie of the devil. I rebuke that lie in Jesus Mighty Name," Michael charged with a rare authority and confidence.

I dropped my head into my hands to hide my tearful emotions. "I can't do this," I squealed aloud. "I'm telling you, I can't do this!" I was afraid of him seeing the weakness of my tears. I had to remain strong, no matter the cost! "I want to see my mother. I need to talk to my mother. Will you take me?" I pleaded.

"Alright, maybe she can make you understand," he said disapprovingly.

"I don't need to understand anything. You need to understand that I don't want another child! How many times do I have to tell you?" I sharply retorted. "Just take me to my mother's," I barked, flinging my purse over my shoulder and walking to the car.

My mother sat at her usual spot in the kitchen, reading a novel. She glanced up at my face, and with her knowing, motherly eyes, she asked, "What's up with you?"

I joined her at the table, lowering my gaze to avoid eye contact for fear that I would break into tears. "I just came back from the doctor," I said as a matter of fact.

"And?... What did she say?" She asked patiently waiting for my response while laying her book aside.

"The doctor diagnosed me with, "Hypoglycemia," or low blood sugar. It is the opposite of Diabetes and there is no medication for it. It is diet controlled carrying the same symptoms as Diabetes such as; insulin shock, coma and death. Simply put, for the first time in my life, I am on a diet," I said sarcastically.

"Your blood sugar is nothing to play around with, Judith," she warned. "What about your tea and soda?" She said, quizzing me.

Like the juice, I figure, if I apply the same principle to my soda, and sip slowly, I can still have at least one a day. I will have to add artificial sugar to my tea, I guess. I am not giving up my sodas," I proclaimed stubbornly.

I drew a deep breath, and said, "Okay, now the really bad news," I said fighting back the tears as I stared out the kitchen window that rested over the dining table. I felt my mother's eyes piercing my face. "The doctor said, it's possible that the baby may be born physically and/or mentally disabled due to the fluctuation of my glucose levels in the past weeks," I said, my voice quivering. I dropping my head into my hands, as the tears welled in my eyes. Everything seemed so surreal. I held my head between my hands, squeezing, attempting to imprison my thoughts to stop them from running amuck. "I don't know what to do," I cried, darting from the table, bouncing against the walls of the long hallway that led to the bathroom. I grabbed a tissue to wipe my eyes and blew my nose. After a short cry, I returned to rejoin my mother.

I covered my eyes as the tears forcefully escaped against my will. My mother handed me a tissue, and pressing her index finger tightly into the table with her fist closed tightly, she firmly stated, "Judith, you need to stay calm. Everything will be alright, you will see," she said with her jaw set firm, nodding her head slightly up and down. "I don't believe it. There is nothing wrong with this baby! The baby will be perfectly healthy. You just watch and see," she affirmed. She held her head in her very own specialized, battle position, as only my mother could do. She poured into me, her inner strength and support that I so grossly needed at that moment.

"No, it's not going to be okay," I murmured. "I didn't want another kid to begin with, and now this? I don't know what to do, mom," I cried. "Michael is always abandoning us for his addictions, and lately, he's been slipping a lot. I don't trust him and I can't carry this load alone. Not anymore," I sniffled and wiped my nose! Another baby is another responsibility, a heavier burden than I'm already carrying, and I just can't do it anymore!"

"What do you think about adoption?" I asked, turning to observe the expression on her face.

"What do you mean?" She asked, puzzled.

"I mean I can't keep this child, Mom. Don't you understand, I am not strong enough to do this alone? I can't," I whimpered full of self-pity. "Why? Why did God do this to me?" I cried in desperation.

"I think it would be better for everyone if I gave the baby up for adoption. Nobody even needs to know," I said.

"What about Michael? What is he going to say?" She asked.

"Michael doesn't need to know yet, and I haven't told him anything either. He doesn't have a say in the matter. He may want another child, but he doesn't want the responsibility that goes with it. He will just leave on his drunken rampages whenever the pressure is on, like he has done for the last seven years," I stated, pessimistically.

My mother lifter her eyes, attempting to fight back her own tears. She wanted to help, but her hands were tied. "You're a grown woman and you're going to do what you're going to do. I can't stop you," she said disappointed. "I don't believe there is anything wrong with this baby, and I won't have it any other way," She commanded.

Michael came in for a glass of water. "Judith, we should go. It's getting close to dinner. Are you ready?" he asked.

We returned home to finish out the day with our silent thoughts.

"C'mon, wake up sleepyhead," Michael said, stroking the side of my face. "It's time to go to the doctor. You are supposed to see the dietician today, remember? I want to stop at the Friday prayer meeting to ask them to pray over you and the baby."

"What if Michael is right, and this is our little girl? Please Jesus, would you help our baby?" I momentarily entertained the idea of a supernatural miracle. No! I don't want another child and I should be able to give up this baby without a hitch. Michael will change his mind once he realizes how difficult it will be to raise it.

"I don't know why God is doing this. Perhaps, He is punishing me for trying to abort the baby. I'm not going to keep the baby, Michael. I've decided to give it up for adoption, unless you want to raise it by yourself. I want the baby to be healthy, so I can find it a good home," I sullenly remarked.

He tilted his head back and I could see the disapproval and disgust in his face. "I'll get the boys ready while you get ready," he announced dejectedly.

Michael told Pastor Browning and Mary Nell about the doctor's concern that the child may be born brain damaged, or physically deformed because of the fluctuation of my blood glucose.

"Oh no! It will not!" Sister Mary Nell exclaimed. Pastor Browning wrung his hands and said, "We will all agree that this baby will be born healthy and strong."

Mary Nell sat at the piano and played as we snuck out to make my appointment on time.

We saw the dietician and returned home to plan our meals in advance. I didn't know how long it would take to get my blood sugar completely under control. I felt embarrassingly inadequate as a whole person, a mother and a wife.

We went in for an ultra sound, after filling my bladder with liquid. "Do you think we can do this fairly quick," I asked the receptionist. "I really have to pee and I don't know if I can hold it much longer," I smiled.

I was immediately taken to the back as I motioned for Michael to join me. A moment later, the technician came in. She smeared a glob of cold gel over my belly and we listened to the machine sound out the baby's heartbeat. We watched the fetus secured in my womb on the monitor.

"Would you like to know the sex of the baby?" The technician asked.

"No," I shouted. "Don't tell me the sex of this baby."

"It's okay. If you don't want to know, I won't tell you. Your secret is safe with me," she said, smiling. "We are finished here. You can get dressed and leave now," she said exiting the room.

I returned the following week to see Dr. Stanheiser. "So far, it all looks good," she said. "The ultra sound didn't show anything out of the ordinary, but you must remember that ultra sounds are not always accurate and it won't tell me anything about the baby's brain. We will have to wait until the baby is born to see what, if any, damage has occurred. Your blood glucose readings are all good. Good job, Judith," she said, encouraging me.

"We just have to stay positive," Michael cheered after returning home. We have to pray, and agree together that God will help us, Judith," his words rung out with faith.

The days passed and I finally found a balance in my glucose levels, and my diet. I felt stronger and more energetic and decided to plant a vegetable garden in the back. I thought the fresh vegetables would keep me healthier, and keep me busy enough to not focus on the pregnancy, that I never wanted to begin with.

After praying and thinking everything through, I didn't believe there was anything wrong with our child. I decidedly believed, God would birth a perfectly healthy, and whole baby from my womb. Michael was so smart, and so handsome, any woman would be truly blessed to adopt this child. I searched the phone book for a local adoption agency, called the number and nervously waited as I listened to the phone ring. I wasn't sure what to do, or what to say, but I couldn't keep this child, and I knew it.

"Riverside County Adoption Services," I heard the woman's voice announce.

"Hello, my name is Judith Birdsong, and I would like to speak with someone about giving my child up for adoption. I am seven months pregnant and already have two children. Financially I can't take on another child," I explained. "Even if I could take financial responsibility, I don't want another child," I told her.

"Hello Judith, my name is Karla. I need some information for our records. Karla, began an inquisition to detail my circumstances and my pregnancy. Who is the father? Where is the father? Who is the doctor? When is your due date? The questioning was endless and tiresome.

Inundated with questions, I was determined to portray the strength of a resolute decision to give up this child.

Karla and I spoke for a period of time. I forfeited the information she requested. I told her that neither the father, nor I had any unresolved issues about giving the child up for adoption. I knew I would have to convince Michael of this, but I didn't' believe he really wanted to be responsible for another child anyway. I didn't want to believe that he would make me keep this baby, knowing full well that he wasn't finished with his drinking sprees.

Karla ended our conversation by telling me that she would research some information for me, and call me back in a few days.

I wasn't sure how Michael would react to the idea of putting our child up for adoption. I justified my actions by telling myself, "I don't even know if he will still be around when I have this baby. He may be out partaking of his drink, or fulfilling one of his sexual fantasies with another woman, when this child is born. Why should he get all the celebratory rights, while I'm left home to carry all the responsibilities," I told myself. "Oh well, I'll deal with it when the time comes."

I returned to the back yard to water my flourishing vegetable garden. Everything was producing in abundance and looking very healthy. I couldn't wait to pick my vegetables and start canning.

Michael returned home looking terribly frazzled from the heat. I smelled the whiskey, realizing his condition was not just the heat, but inebriation.

"You're drunk," I yelled!

He threw his head back, gazing into the open space with his lips pursed as he usually did when confronted about his drinking.

A rage overcame my senses and I felt I had to fight to save whatever was left of my family. "How can I fight a can of beer, or a bottle of whiskey?" I asked myself, as my adrenaline raced through every part of my body.

"You want to destroy our home, here let me help you, Michael," I shouted. I started to throw things across the living room floor. "Why do you keep doing this? I'm pregnant and you want me to keep this child while you run amuck in the bars with other women and get drunk," I screamed while suffocating in the feelings of betrayal. I ran to the kitchen in my rage and threw the melamine dishes. I searched for something more to throw and reached for the glass dishes. The sound of breaking glass shattered into fragments across the floor's surface, as I scathingly shouted, "Sometimes, I hate you, so much!"

I felt something strike the side of my body, sending me reeling across the floor, onto the broken glass that was strewn across the kitchen. I reached out my hands to break my fall, and felt my stomach strike the floor, landing on my side. Sharp pains raced through my belly and I gasped for air as my body contorted into knots underneath me.....

Chapter 5
A SPIRIT OF MURDER

The intensity of fear and rage resonated, violently out of control. I perceived everything around me as my own personal battle to conquer, kill, and destroy the can of beer, or bottle of whiskey, that Michael had been having a lucid affair with over the years. I desperately fought, with every ounce of my being, to save my relationship, Michael, my children, and even my own life. I laid on the floor and my body contorted into knots underneath me. There was pressure in the center of my belly, and a sharp pang pierced through my gut, as I realized Michael was on top of me. I furiously swung my fists and kicked, in an attempt to dislodge his knee that was sharply pressing into the side of my belly. I screamed out, "I swear, Michael! I swear I will kill you if you don't let go and get off of me." I seethed, writhing furiously out of control. "You have to let me up sometime," I screamed venomously.

I struggled to slip out from under his weight that rested on top of me, my eyes piercing his with sheer determination to win the battle. I managed to contort one of my legs, sliding it under his hip as I gave a quick, hard thrust, throwing him off of me breaking his hold on my wrists. I rolled over and sprung to my knees, striking him across his forehead with my fist.

"Stop it, Judith! Just stop it," he demanded clutching my wrists tightly, pinning me down once again. "Get control of yourself. I'm not letting go until you do. You are out of control and you're scaring us," he cried out of his own desperation.

"Okay," I said, relinquishing the battle.

Michael stood to his feet, hurdling a barrage of questions, asking, "Are you hurt? Do you need a doctor? I didn't want to hurt you, Judith. I just wanted to stop you," he said remorseful.

I raised myself from the floor, floating in the remnant of my anger, and noticed several small cuts as a result of falling on the broken glass. Blood was trickling from my wounds and the cuts were stinging my flesh. I reached over for a paper towel to wipe the blood off my arms and hands. Anger consumed me and I didn't know how to let it go. If I fought hard enough, and set an example of sobriety, maybe I could make Michael realize how wonderful life can be sober. Then I could have my husband, and the father of my children back again.

I reached for the broom to clean-up. Michael kept the boys entertained, while I released the remnant of my anger through aggressive cleaning tactics. Angry with God as well as Michael, I yelled, "God, why won't you make him stop drinking, smoking pot, and using drugs?"

Once I finished cleaning, I sat on the sofa reading my bible, and praying for change in our lives. I turned to 2 Peter 2:9 and read,

"Then the Lord knows how to deliver the godly out of temptations and reserve the unjust under punishment for the day of judgment."

"Please Jesus, deliver me from my anger, and Michael from his addictions," I cried out, fighting the doubt and unbelief that encompassed my mind. "Please Jesus, I'm begging, stop him from drinking and give me back the beautiful, intelligent and loving man that I love so much!"

The days were long and hot, and I was growing larger and more uncomfortable. Dr. Stanheiser came into the examining room and determined that I was significantly better. I was learning to recognize the early symptoms to keep my blood glucose under control, although I still had moments of extreme dizziness and vertigo. Learning to regulate and maintain my glucose levels was quite a challenge for me. I struggled daily for the return of some resemblance of normalcy in my life.

"I want to know something Dr. Stanheiser," I said.

"Yes, what is it?"

"You know I never wanted to get pregnant, and I certainly don't want a fourth child. I want to know if you will do a Tubal Ligation the very second I spit this child out.

I don't want to wait one minute longer. I want you to tie my tubes, cut them, burn them, cauterize them, plug them, double knot them, rip them out, or whatever you have to do to make sure I don't ever get pregnant again," I pleaded with my hands folded under my chin.

Dr. Stanheiser laughed and said, "I'll see what I can do. Go home and rest now," she ordered.

We all piled back into the car, where it felt like the fiery furnace of Shadrach, Meshach and Abed-Nego. We drove home with the windows rolled down, becoming ill tempered as the hot desert winds parched our lips and dried our throats. I could hardly wait to get home and drink anything that was ice cold.

I stood in front of the swamp cooler, attempting to cool down and retreated to the sofa when I heard a voice call my name. Sylvia stood at the front door.

"What's going on?" Sylvia inquired. She had been visiting more frequently since her and my younger brother, Daryl, were living together.

At one time, Sylvia, her husband, and Daryl were the closest of friends, and inseparable. Sylvia and Ron had split up, leaving Sylvia and Daryl to couple, becoming an item. Daryl had fallen madly in love with Sylvia and wanted to marry her. I sensed that Sylvia on the other hand, was none too sure of her feelings for Daryl. I knew she loved him, but wondered in what capacity she loved him. For now, Sylvia was married to Ron, who decided she was worth fighting for, and wanted her back. Ron returned to declare Sylvia, his territory and wanted to duel with Daryl to win back his wife.

"I was reading my bible and talking to Jesus," I said. "Michael and the boys are outside playing. Did you leave your boys outside with Michael and the kids?"

"Yeah, she responded. "He is playing catch with them. I was bored and came to visit for a while," she said. We discussed everyday events, our children, and her relationship with Daryl. She complained that her husband was hell bent on breaking them up, and wanted her back. I shared the things God was laying on my heart, and scriptures that were convicting me. I read Matthew 5:27 aloud to her.

"You have heard that it was said to those of old, 'You shall not commit adultery.' "But I say to you that whoever looks at a woman to lust for her has already committed adultery with her in his heart. "If your right eye causes you to sin, pluck it out and cast it from you; for it is more profitable; for you that one of your members perish, than for your whole body to be cast into hell."

I shared the scriptures I had studied, and the guilt I felt for living in sin with Michael. I confided to her, "Michael and I are not legally married, but living together. I have assumed my position as his common law wife, but we are not legally married," I explained. "We are living together in sin. I feel like God wants us to get married, and get our lives right before God," I said, divulging my thoughts. "I am not just a fornicator, but I am an adulterer because I am still legally married to another man. A man I married when I was only nineteen years old. We were together about a month, or so, before separating. He fought, and wouldn't give me a divorce. I thought with time he would come around. Now I can't afford a divorce," I said, disclosing my secrets. Sylvia intently listened, asking an occasional question as we continued the study of adultery. Feeling convicted of my sins, I read Ephesians 5: 3-6,

But, fornication and all uncleanness or covetousness, let it not even be named among you, as is fitting for saints; neither filthiness, nor foolish talking, nor course jesting, which are not fitting, but rather giving of thanks. For this you know that no fornicator, unclean person, nor covetous man, who is an idolater, has any inheritance in the kingdom of Christ and God. Let no one deceive you with empty words, for because of these things the wrath of God comes upon the sons of disobedience.

I shared another scripture in 1 Corinthians 6: 9

Do you not know that the unrighteous will not inherit the kingdom of God? Do not be deceived. Neither

fornicators, nor idolaters, nor adulterers, nor homosexuals, nor sodomites, nor thieves, nor covetous, nor drunkards, nor revilers, nor extortioners will inherit the kingdom of God.

She had been showing an interest in the bible, and in what I was sharing with her. I took advantage of her interest, using every opportunity to minister the word of God to both, Daryl and Sylvia. It wasn't hard to see that God was convicting her heart, as He had been convicting mine. Closing my bible and setting my notes aside, I stood to say good bye to Sylvia.

Over the course of the next few days, Sylvia frequently visited. We were spending a lot more time together and my trust in her increased, bringing us closer to one another.

One afternoon, she came to the door, requesting to speak with me about something that was bothering her. I heard the distress in her voice as she told me she had some questions to ask me.

"Do you remember our conversation about adultery, a few days ago?"

"Of course, I remember," I confirmed, smiling.

"Well, do you think God is going to send me to hell because I am living with Daryl and married to someone else?" Her words trembled with concern and fear.

"Oh, Sylvia," I said in surprise! "I don't know how to answer that, exactly, but Jesus is a loving, forgiving God. The bible says so in Ephesians 1: 7-8,

In Him we have redemption through His blood, the forgiveness of sins, according to the riches of His grace which He made to abound toward us in all wisdom and prudence.

I continued to explicate, using scripture and the facts of life. I reassured her, she was no more going to hell, than I was. I reminded her that Michael and I have been living together for the last seven years. I know we are living in sin, but I also know that Jesus has forgiven us, and He will help us to get ourselves in right standing, according to His word. "Just pray and ask Him to forgive you," I told her.

"Will I have to ask forgiveness for the same thing, every single day? Why can't we just live together and be happy? I don't see what's wrong with it, or why God would send me to hell just for being happy," she said, frustrated.

We reviewed scriptures and the Ten Commandments. I explained to her that we need to ask for forgiveness daily, because we continually sin, falling short of the Glory of God. I reminded her that Jesus shed His blood and died on the cross so we could be forgiven, and live eternally with Him. I gently told her that if God was convicting her heart of sin, she would have to make a choice. "You need to either go back to Ron, or divorce him and marry Daryl. You need to pray about it to make the right decision.

"I will have to think about it," Sylvia replied, deep in thought as she left for home.

The day had been very eventful to say the least. I had fully utilized every opportunity to witness for Christ. "Perhaps, Jesus will use her to witness and lead my brother to Christ," I thought cheerfully.

Excited about watching God work in Sylvia's heart, I pondered on my relationship with my closest friend, Debbie. She was a sister in Christ, and we had been the closest of friends since what seemed to be the beginning of time. We loved each other like family while always helping and supporting one another. Other than my mother, I felt Debbie was the only one I could truly trust and as such, I appointed her my best friend, my confidant, my sister. We had both lived in the South Bay Region of Southern California where we met, until a couple of years ago. Since I moved to the desert, we completely relied on the telephone to bind and sustain our friendship. If we didn't have a phone, it was usually because we talked a little too much. As a result, we would temporarily lose our service, until we managed to pay our bill, reestablishing service, once more.

Sensing that my thinking was getting fuzzy and confused, I started toward the kitchen to snack on some protein. My hands trembled as my blood sugar dropped. The phone rang, and I reached to answer it.

"Hello," I answered, stretching the phone cord to reach the refrigerator, grabbing a block of cheese.

"Hey Judith Woodith, what are you doing? Debbie rang out joyfully.

"Hey, Debbie Webby," I cheerfully sang out, shoving a chunk of cheese into my mouth. "What's going on with you?" I asked apologetically, "Sorry, my mouth is full of cheese, because my blood sugar is acting up," I said, swallowing the cheese to repeat, "What's up with you?"

"Nothing, I just wanted to tell you that I got some money and I'm coming out to see you this weekend," she excitedly squealed into the receiver!

"Really? Oh thank you Jesus," I cried out, indicating my surprise. "I can't wait to see you. Okay, I'll plan dinner for us. I'm pregnant and it's hot, so I can't do very much right now, but we can always sit and visit each other," I said.

"Okay, I have to go now, but I wanted to tell you I'll be there Saturday morning. Woo Hoo!" Debbie hollered in excited pleasure.

Michael returned from work, carrying a beautiful, hand carved, wooden bassinet. I could smell the alcohol on him and knew he had been drinking. I confronted him, and as usual, he denied it. After exchanging a few unpleasant words, we turned our focus back to the bassinet.

"It's beautiful," I commented. "I guess I could make a skirt with a matching blanket and pillow for it," I said.

"That's what I figured. You are very talented, Judith, and I have no doubt, you can clean this old thing up and make it beautiful," he declared, smiling.

I still hadn't told him that I had called the adoption agency. I would wait to call again from the hospital and turn the baby over to them once it was born. Between the fighting and the drinking, I knew I couldn't bring this baby home.

I shared the day's events with Michael. I told him about God convicting Sylvia's heart and how He used me to share with her. "I feel like God is finally using me to minister to others, and it feels really good!" Then I told him that Debbie was coming for the weekend, as he sipped on his iced tea.

"Good, maybe we can barbeque after I get home from work. We'll figure something out," he commented casually, seeing how happy I was.

Saturday morning arrived and I sat down in my rocker teasing the baby, poking it back everywhere it kicked.

The boys ran across the porch, yelling, "She's here! Debbie's here," Jimmy hollered, enthusiastically. Jeffrey pointed toward the road, hollering, "Debbie, Debbie, Debbie," as she entered the gate.

"Yes, we're here," she said, greeting us with a hug. We replenished our overheated bodies with cold drinks, as we conversed about her drive from the L.A. suburbs to the small town of Cabazon. We discussed my due date and she asked what I needed for the baby.

"I have called an adoption agency, and I think I want to give the baby up," I explained. "I haven't told Michael about it yet, so don't say anything," I said rolling my eyes at the thought of telling him. "The adoption agency said I should call them from the hospital, after I have the baby. So, I still have plenty of time to talk to Michael about it."

We spent our time chatting, catching up on everything since we last saw each other. I shared with her about Daryl's new girlfriend, and how God was using me to witness to her.

We broke our conversation to prepare lunch, feed the kids, and send them back outside to play.

Every once in a while, the baby would kick and visibly move around.

"How far along are you?" Debbie asked.

"I'm a little over seven months. The doctor said the baby herniated my belly button, so the baby's feet and hands are really visible whenever it kicks. Excited at seeing the baby kick, Debbie placed her hands on my belly to feel the baby move.

Time flew by and I expected Michael home, soon. The clouds trailed, partially covering the sky to relieve us from the heat that bore down on us in the dry desert terrain.

We reminisced in our memories and experiences, giggling at remembering some of the things we had done.

Suddenly, I heard the front gate slam shut. My ears perked up as I leaned forward to listen for the children playing. The silence rung out in the atmosphere, and I became concerned that the children had left the yard.

I struggled to stand up, lifting myself from the rocker, when I heard a loud thundering noise, clapping against the still atmosphere. It sounded like a gunshot as it echoed loudly throughout the desert floor, and a second time, then a third time.

"Debbie, I'm going to call the kids in, because that sounded like a gunshot to me, and it sounded close," I told her. I started for the front door, concerned for our children's safety, when I was interrupted by a man's voice coming from outside, and in my yard.

"Go get your mom!" I heard Daryl's angry voice shouting at my children.

Puzzled and alarmed, I stepped outside and observed Daryl, holding his rifle. He had taken a stance, holding the gun upright, pointed toward the sky, firing three shots. His jaw was firmly set, his eyes blazed with fury, glaring at me as I approached him. I could see the pure, unadulterated anger, overflowing from his eyes, as they welled up into pools of fire.

"Daryl, what are you doing? Why are you shooting that gun off with my kids in the yard?" I said reprimanding him.

I saw a rage in him that I had never seen before. His words seethed from between his teeth as he yelled, "Where's Michael?"

"You kids get into the house, NOW!" I commanded with an authoritative voice. "Debbie, get the kids inside," I yelled.

Debbie came to the front door and I could see the questioning fear and startled panic shadowing her face with a look of bewilderment. It was as if she were asking, "What is happening here?"

I hollered louder, "Go with Debbie, NOW!"

Debbie called the children by name. They scurried, one by one toward the front door as she quickly guided them indoors and locked the front door behind them. Fear had settled into the air as we wondered what Daryl was doing. Why was he firing his gun and yelling at me?

"Daryl, what's going on? Why are you firing that gun in my front yard? What are you so angry about?" I said waiting for his answer as I walked toward him. I turned my head to glance at the front of the house and saw the children's faces watching out the window. I motioned my hand for them to get out of the window and watched Debbie pull them away, out of the view of the danger that lurked in my front yard.

Without another word, Daryl lost control. He pointed the gun at my belly, moving it slightly up and down, as though it was his finger pointing at me. He shouted hoarsely, "I asked you once, and I won't ask you again. Where is Michael?" He growled with his teeth clenched tightly. "I'm going to kill him! I mean it, Judith! I hate him and I'm going to kill him!"

"He's at work, Daryl," I answered softly, as a protective anger started to rise up inside. "Was he really here to shoot Michael?" I wondered, as multiple questions swarmed my mind all at once.

"Surely, he wouldn't hurt me, on along shoot me, but why was he holding his gun aimed toward my belly?" I would soon be eight months pregnant, surely he wouldn't shoot my unborn child. I contended with my thoughts, convincing myself he meant no real harm. I was becoming increasingly unsure of his intentions with that gun.

I no more than finished my thought, when Daryl deliberately pointed the barrel of the rifle directly in the center of my belly. He firmly held the gun, aimed no more than six inches from my belly button. "I *-x*ing hate him. I am going to kill him and you are not going to have another one of his *-x*ing kids, either. I'm going to kill that *-x*ing kid in your belly," he raged at me.

Again he frothed, "I'll never let you have another one of his *-x*ing kids! If you don't leave him this time, I swear I will kill that b-*$tard in your belly, right now!" The furor behind his venomous sting spilled out and over my heart.

The grown man standing with his gun pointing at my belly was the little brother I had played with, cared for, protected, and loved very much. I stood in disbelief of what I was hearing and seeing. "This is my little brother! This can't be happening!" I was puzzled, confused and shaken, wondering what had happened, causing my brother to behave in such a manner. Horrible visions of my husband and children, shot and killed invaded my mind. I created and imagined multitudes of scenario's that would have made him attack me this way. I couldn't fathom what had happened to make him peculiarly angry enough to kill my husband, and our unborn baby.

The urgency of the confused events caused me to ask again, "What are you so angry about, Daryl?"

He wasn't hearing anything I said, and continued threatening to kill my unborn baby and ordering me to leave my husband. He struck out at me from the depth of his own wounds, pain, and grief as his tears welled up in his eyes, "I hate you, Judith and I hate Michael. I'm not going to let you stay with him. I'm going to kill that b*-x*tard kid of his," he threatened again. Cemented in fury, he continued to scream explicative profanities.

His words continually assaulted me like a brick across my cheek. He vowed to rip my heart out, and hurt me the same way I had hurt him.

"You have destroyed my life, Judith, and now I am going to destroy yours," he said threatening me!

I was confused and frightened by his words. "What did I do to him? I don't understand what I did to hurt him," I thought as my heart raced to seek answers. The confusion settled deeper into my spirit, my own pain and fears were beginning to turn to pure, unadulterated anger, merging with his anger.

It didn't take long before my own worldly, protective emotions entered into the battle. Threatened, for a brief moment I lost my focus and forgot who I was in Christ.

Infuriated, I moved into the barrel of the rifle, pressing it hard against my belly. I slowly moved forward, with the rifle still in his hand, inching him backward with my belly, as I stepped in.

"You had better pull that trigger, Daryl, and when you do, you better d*$mn well make sure you kill me. Because if you don't, I'm going to take that gun away from you, and use it on you," I vowed while elevating my angry, controlled voice. My eyes locked with his, exchanging an intense fiery rage. I let him know I meant business and hoped one of us wasn't going to have to die today.

My sites were locked on Daryl when out of nowhere, somebody unexpectedly grabbed my arm from behind and violently jerked me away from the gun, throwing me off balance.

I was sharply aware of a woman standing in front of me. I broke free of Sylvia's grip and turned back toward Daryl, who was still holding his gun, in time to see my step father, George step between the barrel of Daryl's gun and myself. He reached for the gun and pulled the tip of the barrel upward. Daryl and his father each struggled for possession of the gun, maintaining a firm grip.

I stepped into Sylvia and shoved her back away from me. She took another step back, raising her arms as if to surrender, and said, "Please don't do anything stupid, Judith. He is going to shoot you and kill your baby!"

Standing firm, I positioned my body to fight, realizing this was not the voice of Sylvia, but her twin sister, Sandy.

"I don't care! Somebody tell me what the hell is going on here," I snapped at her!

I glanced watchfully around me, researching my changing surroundings. George continued to struggle with

Daryl, attempting to take the gun from his hands. The situation was escalating to a deadly violence.

George and Daryl held tightly to the rifle with both hands, twisting, tugging, and pulling against each other, thrashing about, each one trying to remove the gun from the other. George was gaining momentum, pushing Daryl back through the gate.

I continued to nervously dance, turning and twisting to watch my surroundings to safeguard and protect myself, and my family. I would be certain nobody would take me by surprise again.

George held firmly to the gun, shouting directives at Daryl, as a father reproving his son.

I worried the gun would discharge in the struggle and accidently shoot somebody.

Sandy blurted, "Sylvia broke up with Daryl a couple of hours ago. She told him she was going back to her husband. He is hurt and very angry," she said. "Sylvia was concerned he was going to do something really stupid and called me. I asked George to help me," she said.

"What does this have to do with me, Michael, or our baby?" I spit angrily.

"He blames you for Sylvia breaking up with him. He said Michael bought some pot from him and promised to pay him when he got his check. He never did pay him and ripped him off. Daryl is mad at everyone right now," she stated.

I pushed Sandy toward the gate, yelling for everyone to get off my property.

The devils name that day was, Chaos, and he was standing right in front of me! I rebuked every evil thing and watched as George gained possession of the gun.

Just then, I heard Michael pull up behind Daryl's car and the struggle for the gun started again.

"Michael, he has a gun and he's going to shoot you! Don't get out of the car. Drive away, right now," I yelled.

Michael drove around the corner and fear overcame my senses as my adrenaline took over.

Once Michael was out of sight, George shoved Daryl into his vehicle and returned the gun to him. Daryl stood the gun up in the car seat, beside him and sped away.

"You okay?" George asked me.

"I don't understand! Sandy told me that Sylvia broke up with him, and he is blaming me," I said mystified.

"I don't know what happened, but I'll find out," George said with his hands thrust deep into the pockets of his light blue, weaved pants. George and I stood in the yard when Michael ran through the gate yelling, "What happened here?"

We briefly explained before George left to return home. Michael and I went inside where I fell into my rocker, exhausted. I described, in more detail to Michael what happened.

Debbie, who had been shaken, confided that she didn't feel safe and wanted to return home. I apologized to her and her children and we said good bye. The phone rang and Michael walked her out while I answered the phone. My mother's strained voice spoke into the phone and asked, "Are you okay?"

She called to tell me that she had calmed Daryl down for the evening, and didn't expect any more problems.

"Sylvia broke up with Daryl and used you as an excuse, Judith. Sylvia said, you told her to break up with Daryl and return to her husband, or she would go to hell," my mother explained. "You need to lay down and rest now. I love you, and I'll call you later," she said before hanging up the receiver.

Michael came in and saw I was upset again. I told him about the conversation I had with my mother. "Apparently, I am to blame for her ending their relationship. I appreciate Sylvia's decision but I don't' understand why she lied about what I said, and didn't say to blame me for this," I said expressing my frustration and anger.

Chapter 6
A CHILD IS BORN

The days passed quietly, since Daryl's violent tirade. In his anger, Daryl continued to act out, with small vengeful actions, attempting to make me pay for his pain. One morning, I told Mary Nell about the quandary that one of his deeds had left us in and requested prayer for his salvation and healing. The church prayed for Daryl in agreement. Mary Nell spoke out with tongues, and silence fell as the crowd awaited an interpretation, and this is what we heard;

"Do not fear for this young man, for I have claimed him as my own dear son, and he will soon be with me."

The Lord had spoken! I left the church in blessed elation, feeling confident Jesus was going to save my little brother, and restore our relationship.

I was nearing my ninth month and went in to see Dr. Stanheiser again.

"I hear you are experiencing some cramps?" She said, looking over my chart, and examining me.

"Well, you are dilated to about two centimeters! It looks like you have started labor, Judith. The baby has dropped and the head is right there, at the opening. I'm guessing, but I think it is possible that when its time, you will deliver in ten to 15 minutes," she said, concerned. I want you to go home and stay completely off your feet. It's too early for the baby to come.

"Are you kidding me? I have two boys and a husband. I can't just lay around," I gasped in surprise!

She gave me a look that told me I wasn't going to win this argument. She proceeded to educate me on the dangers of a premature birth and sent me home.

I drove home with my thoughts swirling in waves of confusion. I really wanted to keep this baby, if only Michael would get sober and act like a responsible husband and father. My heart was softening and I quickly jerked myself back to reality." I can't think like this! I have to set my mind on adoption," I told myself.

I walked into the house to hear Jimmy and Jeffrey screaming, "Mommy's home! Mommy's home! Can we have ice cream now?" I walked into the kitchen to dish some ice cream and flippantly hollered, "I'm in labor!"

"What? Why aren't you in the hospital? Why didn't you call me?" Michael ranted nervously, moving toward me.

"I am only two centimeters, I explained. The doc wants me to stay off my feet, if not in bed to prevent premature delivery and stop the labor, avoiding any further complications for both, myself and the baby. That means you will have to carry the burdens of the home, which means; the kids, gardening, cooking, cleaning and the likes. Will you be okay with that?" I was concerned that the pressure would cause him to relapse into drinking again.

"Of course, I can handle that. I'll do whatever it takes to be sure you and the baby are healthy and safe. I love you Judith, and I love our baby," he whispered, leaning over and snuggling his cheek against my belly.

Michael rose up every morning, made breakfast, watered the garden, and left for work after laying me on the sofa and giving the boys instructions to care for me. In the evening, Michael would return home from work, to make dinner, do dishes and team up with the boys to complete the household chores.

Weeks passed while we continued in our newly established, temporary routine.

I laid on the sofa, giving directives to the boys and Before I knew it, the afternoon came and went. Evening approached and Michael was late returning home. I called the restaurant and was told he left a couple of hours earlier.

"Oh my God," I thought as my heart sank and my adrenaline rushed over me. "I'm pregnant and he has taken off again. He has left me miles from nowhere and taken our only transportation! What am I going to do?" I considered the various options with my mind racing for answers. "He could be anywhere out there, but where?" I asked, my heart swimming in self-pity.

I put the boys to bed and sat on the sofa, sobbing and praying. "Why can't you make him stop drinking, Lord? I am trying so hard to be a good mother, and a good wife," I said, convulsively gasping for my next breath, as I drifted off to sleep.

I awoke the next morning wondering where he could be. 'There are so many places he frequented to drink, from L.A., Temecula, Hemet, Aguanga or even locally," I thought. I wondered if he had lost his job again.

"That's it!" I exclaimed excitedly. "Today is his day off but it is also payday. He will be at the restaurant at 3:00 to pick up his check.

The boys and I walked to my mother's house. I explained my situation and asked to borrow her car to fetch Michael back home.

I pulled into the restaurant parking lot just in time to see Michael starting his engine to leave. I was sure he had seen me since he appeared to be in a rush. Placing both feet in position for the clutch and accelerator, I yelled to the boys, "Hang on," as I accelerated speedily, aiming the center of my mother's car for a head on collision with that old Mercury. Realizing I was not going to back down, he slammed on his brakes, bringing the car to a screeching halt.

I slammed on my brakes, stopping the car just inches from striking the Mercury. I got out of the car holding my belly, and ran to Michael's window screaming, "You want to go party with your friends? Really, Michael? You may not care that I'm in labor, but I do! I didn't get pregnant by myself and I'm not going through this by myself, Michael," I cried out in a fiery rage. I ordered his friends out of our car and demanded that he return home immediately. "How can you do this to our kids, to me, to our baby? The baby you say you want so much? What is wrong with you?" I continued to rant as his friends exited our car while cursing at me for spoiling their party.

"Okay, Okay, I'm sorry, Judith," Michael shamefully said. "I'll follow you back home," he told me.

"No! I'll follow you to my mother's house, and you can drive us back home. Don't even think about trying to get away from me, because I swear, I will hunt you down, Michael," I vowed.

I followed him to my mother's house to return her keys and rode home with Michael and the boys. "I may have to go the hospital, because of all this," I impetuously threatened.

I laid on the sofa, timing my contractions as Michael explained that he left because he couldn't handle all the pressure. Then he dropped the bombshell on me. "I got caught drinking on the job, and I was fired yesterday. I was too ashamed to tell you, so I just kept going. It's not an excuse, just the truth," he said.

"I can't do this alone or without you, Michael," I proclaimed. Well, there is nothing we can do about your job now. Maybe you should take a few days to chill, and pull yourself together. I am ready to pop this baby out any day now, anyway. It's just a matter of when the baby decides to come, or the doctor decides to induce. I will ask her, next time I see her. I have to rest now. I'm too exhausted to talk anymore," I said, closing my eyes.

Evening approached and my labor pains steadied at five minutes apart. "I need for you to take me to the hospital now," I told Michael. We gathered the children, along with our packed bags and loaded the car.

We dropped the boys off with my sister, Debbie, who was just younger than me, by a couple of years. She took in the boys, and we continued on to the hospital.

I rested in the maternity ward, hooked to monitors and waited for the doctor.

Dr. Stanheiser came in, and looked over the monitor results. She said "The baby's head is right there, ready to pop right out. However, you are still only dilated to two centimeters and your contractions are irregular again. You are having what we call, "False Labor," she explained.

"False Labor?" I questioned her diagnosis. "It doesn't feel false to me! It is definitely pain, I feel it and there is nothing false about it! It hurts," I complained.

"Yes it does. The pain may be real, but the baby has no intention of coming out right now. I would guess this baby will deliver in ten to fifteen minutes, once you start to dilate further, but we are in no hurry for this to happen," she said. "Do you live close to the hospital? If not, I would suggest you stay with a family member, or friend who does, from this point on," she warned.

Michael and I discussed where we should stay as we drove to Debbie's to pick up the boys. "Maybe you should ask Debbie if we can stay with her, since they live in Banning," he suggested.

We knocked on Debbie's door, who looked surprised when she saw me standing in front of her. I told her what Dr. Stanheiser said, and asked if we could stay with her until my contractions regulated.

We made a pallet for the boys, on the floor of her living room, beside the hide-a-bed that we made out for ourselves.

After a couple of days, we realized the inconvenient burden we had placed on my sister and agreed to return home, trusting God that all would turn out well.

It had been more than a month since Dr. Stanheiser first told me I had dilated two centimeters. Michael had been jonesing for a drink, and I became a nervous wreck, not knowing if he was going to stick around or not. I caught him sneaking out the gate to leave, twice since returning from my sisters. I felt the urge to follow him everywhere he went. I fearfully treaded on egg shells, every time I saw him walk toward the front door. I did everything I could to relieve him of any pressure or excess burdens.

I had been making three to four trips a week to the hospital, with regular contractions. It followed that every time I checked in, my labor pains became irregular again. "Another false alarm," was quickly becoming the new by-word used to describe this birth. I became more and more frustrated, just wanting it to be over with, so I could call the Adoption Agency to pick up the baby. I wanted to be free from the burden of fear and torment that heavily weighed on me.

Once again, I laid in the small examining room, with Dr. Stanheiser. Before she was able to speak, I plead with her, "Please, please, please induce my labor now. I just want to have this baby. I can't take it anymore," I cried in misery

She smiled, and said, "If you haven't had it in the next few days, I will induce on October first," she replied. "You can take it for just one more week, can't you? You will need to check into maternity at 5:00 a.m. on the first of October. I will induce at 6:00 a.m. and you should deliver by 6:05, and it will be over with," She said with a giggle. "I know you are frustrated, but I want to give this baby a chance to gain more weight," she insisted.

I returned to the waiting area to tell Michael of the plan to induce on the first of the month, if I hadn't given birth by then. A smile spread across both of our cheeks as we journeyed home.

Over the course of the final week, we had made two more trips to the hospital, only to hear the infamous words, "Another false alarm!" It was obvious that the baby was being stubborn in its decision, to not come out and greet the world.

The alarm sounded at 4:00 a.m. Finally, it was time to go to the hospital. We left the boys with my sister the night before in preparation of our early morning start. I still hadn't told Michael about the adoption, for fear he would be angry. I decided I would spring it on him after the child was born.

Michael carried my bag to the car and we started out for the hospital.

We arrived at San Gorgonio Memorial Hospital at 4:55 a.m. I laid in the delivery room, watching the monitors while Michael held my hand, standing beside me.

At 6:10 a.m. Dr. Stanheiser entered my room to inject my I.V., instructing the nurse to watch me closely.

"It won't be long now," she said, exiting the room.

The contractions increased, getting much stronger, and quicker. I moaned and Michael coached my breathing.

"You can push anytime now," Dr. Stanheiser announced as she lowered herself to a "Johnny Bench" position. "Okay, push," she ordered.

Michael joined her at my feet, for a birds eye view of the birth of our baby.

"I'm guessing this baby is a girl, weighing exactly five and a half pounds, what about you?" Dr. Stanheiser asked the attending nurse.

"An even five pounds," the nurse responded, when the grandmother of all birthing pains hit me.....

"Ayyyyyyeeeeee," I screamed as loudly as I could, blacking out momentarily.

Dr. Stanheiser lifted the baby over the sheets for me to see her, calling out, "Just as I thought, it's a girl!"

"It's a girl? A girl? Oh my God, let me see," I said, exhausted. "Please, let me see her! It's a girl," I cried out. This was my baby, my little girl. Nothing mattered anymore, she was my little girl, and I loved her. She was mine," I thought. "I love her despite every circumstance, every hardship, and every obstacle. Disregarding every attempt I had made, not to love her, I loved her anyway. She is my precious daughter, my precious baby girl, and I would never give her up. It doesn't matter to me if she is perfect, or healthy, or not. I love her and she is mine.

"Here daddy," she said to Michael, handing him our baby. "You want to help clean her up," she said, instructing him to lay her on the scale. "She is five pounds, eight and one half ounces, and arrived at 6:39 a.m. I was only half an ounce off this time," she declared, giggling.

Our baby girl was perfect. She had all ten fingers and toes, and she is incredible. Michael returned with our little Jeni-lee, cleaned, dressed, and beautiful.

"Okay, we are taking you to your room now. Someone will be in shortly to take you to surgery. I will see you then," Dr. Stanheiser informed me.

I was transferred to my room. I no more than hit the sheets, before another nurse came in to put me back on a gurney, taking me to O.R.

I awoke that afternoon to the sound of a television in my room. I quickly realized the pain in my body as I struggled to move myself. The nurse came in and injected me with a pain reliever leaving me drowsy and I quickly drifted off to sleep.

I awoke to Dr. Stanheiser standing over me. She told me that everything went well in surgery, she had repaired my herniated belly button, and the Tubal Ligation was a great success.

"Well, Judith, I did everything you asked me to do. I cut your fallopian tubes, tied them in double knots, cauterized them, plugged them, and did everything but rip them out," she said, laughing. Suddenly she quit laughing and with a very stern look, she warned me, "If you should get pregnant again, don't you dare come to see me," she said laughing at her declaration of non-responsibility.

A few minutes later, Michael stumbled into my room, handing me a small bouquet of roses and leaned over to kiss me. Revolted by his breath that reeked of whiskey, I pushed him away from me.

"They're beautiful, thank you honey," I said and scolded him for getting drunk. "Getting drunk is not the way to celebrate the birth of our beautiful daughter," I told him. "Aren't we a pair, you drunk and me loaded on pain medicine," I proclaimed.

"Judith, I'm sorry, he said, cocking his head back, avoiding eye contact as he did every time he drank. "My friends wanted to buy me a celebratory drink when I passed out the cigars. I couldn't say no, I'm sorry," he said with little or no regret. He smiled as his eyes lit up in a way I had not seen for a very long time. The tears of joy welled, in his beautiful brown eyes.

"The hospital has sibling visitations every afternoon. Maybe tomorrow you can bring the boys. I can't seem to stay awake," I told him drifting off once again.

My roommates husband came to visit her, shortly after I had awoke. He told me, he had seen my little girl in the nursery. "She is really a beautiful baby. I just wish my wife would have given me a pretty baby like yours," he sarcastically spewed at her, leaving me stunned. He left the hospital and his wife cried, leaving me to comfort her.

"Your baby is just as beautiful as mine," I said, when another couple entered my room.

"We saw your baby in the nursery and wanted to tell you that she is probably the most beautiful baby we have ever seen," they said complimenting me gracefully.

My baby girl was becoming a hospital celebrity. I recalled years before, thinking, if Michael and I had a little girl, she would be the most beautiful little girl in the world, and now it has come to pass. We did have the most beautiful little girl in the world, and I loved her more than life!

The three days in the hospital passed quickly and Michael took me home with our newest edition to the family, our beautiful Jeni-lee.

My sister, Debbie greeted us at her front door and with one fell swoop, she took Jeni-lee from my arms, kissing her little face and coddling her in her arms. Jimmy and Jeffrey ran excitedly, locking their arms around me, yelling, "Mommy!"

"Be careful, mommy has a really big "owie," on her tummy," Michael cautioned the boys. The boys let go of me and stood gazing at their new little sister.

It was our first night home and a persistent cough stirred me from my sleep. I sat up to spit some phlegm into a Kleenex. In the darkness, I saw something dark against the white tissue. I turned the light on to see what it was, when I noticed a significant amount of blood in the tissue. I awakened Michael to ask him what I should do.

"I am going to call Dr. Stanheiser. I don't care if it is one in the morning," he said.

The answering service contacted Dr. Stanheiser, who returned our phone call moments later. She asked the color of the blood, and Michael told her it was brown.

"The anesthesia in surgery caused some bleeding in her lungs because of smoking," she told me. "Just relax, if it is brown, then it is old blood and will clear up in time. If it becomes red again, immediately go to the ER," she said before hanging up.

Morning came and Michael fed Jeni-lee, allowing me to sleep in after a rough night of coughing. He lifted her cradle, moving it to the living room. The boys who were usually up by now and crying for breakfast, remained in their beds.

He went in to wake the boys, shaking their shoulders and singing "Bullfrogs and Butterflies" aloud. Jimmy looked up and whimpered with a small voice, "Daddy, I don't feel good." Then, Jeffrey chimed in, "I sick daddy!"

Michael felt their foreheads and discovered they were both running fevers. He asked, "Where don't you feel good?"

Both the boys put their hands on their throats and murmured, "My throat hurts, daddy."

Laying both the boys on a pallet in the living room, he came to tell me that we had two sick little boys. I sat on the bed shaking, cold, and speaking nonsensical gibberish, when he realized that I was also delirious with fever. He carried me to the pallet, laying me next to the boys.

Michael and the boys returned from the pediatrician a few hours later with a diagnosis of strep throat. The doctor had prescribed enough medication for all of us, except Jeni-lee, whose immune system still protected her.

The weeks passed and Jeni-lee was nearly three months old. She was in perfect health, very alert, and was growing quickly.

"Michael, come look at your daughter!" I hollered for him to come watch her stand freely on my lap, with her tiny little hands gripping my index fingers. "She is going to be an early walker. You can mark my words," I vocalized.

The following morning I lifted Jeni-lee from her crib to check her, concerned with her cough and fussing. She was terribly warm so I took her temperature. The thermometer read 103 F. After administering Tylenol, she became very lethargic and I had trouble waking her. She was refusing nourishment and liquids.

"We need to take her to the ER, Michael. I can't explain it, but this just doesn't feel right to me. I have a really bad feeling," I expressed fretfully.

The children's pediatrician, Dr. Lennox, came into the examining room and said Jeni-lee had pneumonia. He prescribed her some antibiotics and said I could take her home.

"No," I exclaimed! "I'm sorry Dr. Lennox, I can't explain it, but I'm afraid to take her home. I live out in Cabazon and her breathing is too erratic. What if she needs emergency care and we can't get here in time? I have a bad feeling about this. Can't you keep her here until she is better?" I said, pleading with him.

Sympathetic to my fears, Dr. Lennox hesitated, then agreed to admit Jeni-lee for a couple of days, to run tests and observe her.

I remained at the hospital with her until about 10:00 that evening, until she fell asleep. I was sure she would sleep through the night and left for home with the intention of returning before she awoke in the morning.

I woke before Michael, dressed and returned to the hospital by 5:30, in the wee morning hours.

I was shocked, and fear immersed my heart when I saw Jeni-lee in her metal barred crib, which was completely covered in a plastic sheet, pumping oxygen into the tent. She was laying on her back, devoid of any color and her limbs were strapped to the bars of the crib. There was an I.V. needle inserted in the top of her head.

"Dear Jesus, what happened to my baby girl?" I cried out in a panic. I dropped my purse and swiftly ran to the nurse's station.

"What happened to my baby?" I yelled to the nurse. She walked me back to Jeni-lee's room and said, "Your baby took a turn for the worse in the night. We tied her down so she couldn't tear the I.V. needle loose. She is stabilized for now. The doctor will be in soon to explain further," she said before returning to the nurse's station.

I immediately called Michael to tell him what had happened. He took the boys to a sitter and joined me at the hospital where we waited together for the doctor.

Dr. Lennox entered a short time later. He explained that her fever had spiked during the night. He told us, she had the croup, and was borderline pneumonia. He had ordered aspirin to be administered both, rectally and intravenously to bring her fever down.

"She is showing great improvement and I will probably send her home this afternoon, if she continues to show this kind of progress," Dr. Lennox said.

Michael was excited, and I was very reluctant to take her home, but I didn't understand why. "I don't want to take her home, Michael. I can't explain it, but I know there is something very, very wrong. I'm asking you to trust me. I have a really bad feeling." I said trying to convince him that I was right.

Michael, in no uncertain words, let me know that I was an overly protective, paranoid mother. Of course, I became defensive and we squabbled, right then and there.

Dr. Lennox returned to the room and I argued with him about his decision to release her. He insisted, he could not find a valid reason to keep her any longer.

I was angry with Dr. Lennox for not believing, or trusting my motherly instincts. I knew something was terribly wrong with my daughter. Realizing there was nothing more I could do, and having no say in the matter, I packed up my daughter and headed for home.

I made a pallet in the center of our large wooden spool that had been stained and lacquered, serving as a coffee table. I laid Jeni-lee down on the pallet in front of me and said, "I don't care what anyone thinks, I am not taking my eyes off of her, not for a minute," I declared.

I planted myself on the sofa and watched her very closely, never leaving her side as I watched TBN on the television.

I prayed asking Jesus to show me why I was having this feeling, and my gut kept telling me not to take my eyes off of Jeni-lee. I took her temperature every 15 to 30 minutes throughout the day. Each time, it read 98.6. I still couldn't shake the feeling of dread and doom that loomed over me as I observed her into the evening hours and through the night.

Morning came and the boys traipsed down the long hallway, and into the living room, rubbing their sleepy little eyes, searching for their breakfast.

I poured their cereal and made a pot of coffee for Michael before waking him.

"Its 7:00 sleepy head," I said stroking his shoulder. Michael, I've been up all night, and I'm exhausted. Would you please watch Jeni-lee while I take a short nap? I won't nap for very long, I promise," I begged with my eyes half shut.

"I fed the boys and made your coffee. She is okay right now, I just need for you to keep a close eye on her for me," I begged.

After a couple of minutes of stretching, he moved to sit in front of Jeni-lee. I gave him, his coffee and instructions. Whatever you do, don't fall back asleep, take her temperature every 15 minutes, watch her and wake me up in two hours," I said, retiring to my bed for a quick wink.

Thirty minutes into my sleep, I heard a deep voice hollering my name. I looked up to see Michael's fear filled expression as he stood over me.

"Judith, something is really wrong with Jeni-lee. I don't know what to do," he said urgently.

I reacted with instant panic, standing to my feet at the foot of the bed and with one forceful leap into the living room, I stood beside her pallet. Instantly, I knew something was very wrong. My worst fears had manifested, standing uncovered before my very eyes and revealed itself in its fullness.

In a split second, my entire life had just changed. Her eyes had rolled into the back of her head, and all I could see were the whites of her eyes. I quickly observed her arms contorted, and twisted. They were drawn up, behind her, crisscrossed and locked in the center of her back. Her knees were bent and drawn, nearly to her chin as her tiny lower legs tried to wrap themselves along the side of her body. Her back was severely arched and her head was thrown back behind her. Her neck was so severely contorted and twisted that her head lay cocked almost between her shoulder blades.

I reached over to pull on her leg gently, attempting to straighten her, only to realize she was locked into an unmovable position. Her flesh felt like she was on fire, her mouth was agape and there were small, delayed, shallow thrusts coming from her lungs that sounded like each breath would be her last. There was a gurgle in her throat with every breath she fought to inhale, reminding me of the death rattle. I wondered if that was what I was witnessing now. I grabbed the thermometer, yelling at Michael, "How long has she been like this?"

"It just happened when I woke you up, Judith. Is she going to be okay? What's wrong with her?" Michael asked, looking to me for answers.

I placed the thermometer against her and it instantly shot to 106 F, the limit of the thermometer. "I don't know," I yelled running back to the bedroom to slide into my dirty pants from the top of the hamper. I grabbed the hem of my full length nightgown, pulling it up and knotting it at my waist.

The small town of Cabazon, still had no paramedic service. Realizing the nearest help was stationed in Hemet,

I pulled the blankets over my daughter, lifted her from the pallet and screamed, "In Jesus Mighty Name, you will not die!"

With my strongest commando voice, I yelled, "Michael, let's go now! Grab the boys and get in the car, right now!

Michael called to the boys, "Get dressed quick!"

"No," I yelled fiercely. There is no time to waste! We will all go to the hospital just as we are. Get in the car this minute," I yelled again.

We rushed to the car as I held Jeni-lee against my heart, praying for her life. Michael drove 55 mph along the baron wasteland of the lonely desert road.

"Michael, our baby is about to take her last breath! She is going to die in my arms if you don't speed up and get us there. You better drive a lot faster, or pull over and you can hold her while I drive," I yelled distressed and consumed with fear for my daughter's life.

Michael sped up and we arrived at the ER in minutes. I leapt from the car with bare feet and my baby in arms. I approached the front station screaming, "Something is wrong with my baby, she's not breathing!"

I fought back the tears as a nurse ran toward me. She led me to an examining table and I asked for Dr. Lennox. The nurse said he was out of town for the weekend, and was unreachable.

Doctors and nurses came in and out of the ER examining room, calling STAT. I heard the attending doctor order aspirin to be administered rectally, and told the nurse they needed take whatever measures necessary, to bring her fever down.

The doctor returned, ordering tests for Jeni-lee. He suspected Spinal Meningitis was the culprit behind this. Suddenly, I could hear my own heart beating and panic manifested as I heard one nurse tell another, she was tending an infant who had just been coded.

I turned to the doctor, "Is she going to be okay? Is my baby going to die?" I asked, barely able to speak the words.

"I can't say at this point. Your baby is seriously ill. I will do everything medically possible, but I can't tell you she will be okay, not just yet," he said compassionately.

I dropped my head into my hands and cried, "Jesus, please help my baby girl!"

"I have ordered a spinal tap, and will rush the lab for results. I should have all the test results back very soon. Hopefully we will know more soon and I will see you again in a little bit," the doctor told me before walking away.

I turned toward the nurse and said, "I'll be right back. I need to go to the waiting room and tell my family what is going on."

I swiftly walked to the waiting room, where Michael and the boys had been patiently waiting for news about Jeni-lee. I saw the heaviness of concern on Michael's face. The boys played on the floor quietly, next to him.

"Michael," I called his name aloud. He leapt from his chair to approach me for answers.

I fought for composure as I explained that Jeni-lee was on the critical list and coded. "They don't know if she will be okay, or not," I said tearfully.

We discussed the crisis and I asked Michael to take the boys to a sitter and contact Pastor Browning for prayer. Then, I asked him to please, bring me back some clean clothes, a toothbrush, and a pair of shoes.

I returned to the ER and continued to pray, binding every evil thing, and sealing myself up in my spiritual armor, even though I didn't completely understand the armor part, or how it worked.

"My daughter will be healed, and she will be fine," I proclaimed aloud in faith. I was in a mindset that said, "Nothing, but nothing shall conquer Christ Jesus, who lives in me, because I believe!"

Suddenly, the fear left me and a righteous anger consumed me. My claws were out, my fangs were showing, and I was ready to battle to the death. "God help any person, demon, or thing that got in my way now." I whispered aloud as I approached my daughter's bed. I laid my hands upon her tiny heart, and proclaimed her healing aloud.

A technician entered the room, and said he was from imaging. He took my daughter to run tests that were ordered by the doctor.

The nurse said, "We will be admitting your daughter to pediatrics. We are going to take some x-rays and do a lumbar puncture, or you may have heard it called a spinal tap. We will also do a lab work-up. It may be best if you wait for your daughter in her room."

I watched them roll Jeni-lee away as the nurse said, "Follow me, I'll take you to her room."

I turned to follow after her and said, "My husband will be returning soon. Will you tell him where we are?"

"Of course," she replied, leaving me alone in the empty, sterilized room, with the atmosphere swirling with the familiar hospital odors.

I sat in a chair next to the cold, steel crib and continued to pray. "Jesus, please help my baby girl and heal her. I don't believe for one minute, that you gave me this precious little girl, made me keep her and love her, despite everything we've gone through, just to take her away from me like this," I sighed grievously.

A nurse came in to tell me I had a phone call at the nurse's station.

I followed her to the phone, picked up the receiver and answered, "Hello."

Whispering with a broken voice, I heard my mother say, "Judith, I just heard." Her voice crumbled as the tears slipped from her eye lids and she wept. "I am coming to the hospital. I'll be there in a few minutes."

"Mom!" I firmly said aloud, "Listen to me! My little girl is going to be fine, in Jesus name! I don't want you to come here if you are going to cry. Don't cry!" I commanded. "I love you mom, but I have to be strong and I won't have tears, or doubt around me right now. I am strong in Christ Jesus, and my little girl is going to be just fine," I said, clearly enunciating every word before hanging up.

A short time later, Michael returned with my clothing. I popped into the bathroom and quickly dressed myself. When I came out fully dressed, I updated Michael.

He told me he had called both our mother's and went to the church to tell them what happened, then asked for prayer. "They are praying and send their love. They are very concerned, Judith," he said, conveying their love to me.

My mother arrived as Jeni-lee returned to her room. I leapt to the nurse's side, asking if they knew anything yet.

"No, not yet," she responded. "The doctor is rushing the lab for results. He will be in to speak with you shortly. We are attempting to stabilize her and get her fever down. So far, we've not been able to get her fever below 105 F. Her respirations are still shallow and decreased," she explained.

"It all happened so fast, I told my mother. I only left her for 30 minutes before Michael woke me. She was fine until I left her," I told my mother, fighting the tears.

"It's not your fault, Judith," she said. "I have to go to work now. Call me if there is any change, no matter how big, or how small. I will leave work and come back here if you need me to. I love you," she said, walking away.

I suggested that Michael leave too. "There is nothing else you can do here. I will stay with her and call you if there is any change."

Minutes after Michael left, a man came in wearing a white coat, pushing a cart with a covered tray on top. He stopped at the side of Jeni-lee's crib. Suddenly, everything became so surreal. I watched as he slipped his gloves on, uncovered the tray and inspected the exposed instruments that were neatly contained therein. I saw him lift a scalpel from the tray to inspect it closely and turned toward my daughter to lift her chin, inspecting her neck.

"What are you doing?" I yelled, lunging to my daughter's side.

"She is very critical. I am here to make sure she continues to breathe and I will be staying with her until she is stabilized," he said firmly.

Realizing he was talking about a tracheotomy, and knowing that I couldn't watch this, I said, "I'm going to the cafeteria and I'll be back shortly," I said helplessly.

"No, you need to stay with your baby," he called out.

"I am not going to stand here and watch you slit my daughter's throat! I understand you are doing what you have to do, to save my daughter, but I am her mother and I will protect her," I said threatening him. "Now, I am going to the cafeteria, if you should need me, you can find me there."

I stopped at the pay phone outside the cafeteria, to call Michael and update him.

Michael returned to the hospital that evening, and together, we sat beside our daughter, agreeing in prayer for her healing. The doctor came in to confirm that Jeni-lee did not have Spinal Meningitis.

"However, she is still running a high fever. We don't have a handle on it, or a diagnosis yet, but I am hopeful that we will know something very soon," he assured us before continuing his rounds.

Morning came, and I was exhausted, sore, and I ached, from sleeping in the chair. I decided to venture off to the cafeteria, in search of a large cup of hot tea.

I returned to Jeni-lee's room to see her legs were pulling upward to her chest. I realized she was starting to seizure again, and ran for a nurse. She said they would have to lay her in ice, because nothing else was working. She left the room and returned with several large buckets of ice, filling the tub and adding cold water to the ice. She left the room and said another nurse would come in to bathe Jeni-lee.

It seemed a long time since the nurse left and nobody returned leaving me alone, anxious and fearful.

When the nurse finally returned, she asked me to put Jeni-lee in the ice. She explained they were very short handed and didn't have anyone available, because it seemed, all the babies needed attention at the same time this morning.

I wasn't sure I could do it.

"We are out of time and we don't have any choices left, we have to get her fever down immediately," she said, compelling me to lay Jeni-lee down in the tub of icy water.

I held Jeni-lee's naked body in my arms, with her bare, burning flesh searing into my own flesh. I drew her protectively against my body, walking to the tub filled with water and crushed ice. The heat radiated from her body as it would from a fireplace, and I immersed her body into the icy cold water.

I watched her muscles tighten as the icy cold water assaulted her hot flesh. She screamed aloud and the shock of the cold struck her, like a fist striking a heavy blow to her belly.

I completely submerged her, all but her little face. This was the first time I heard her cry since the whole ordeal began. She continued to scream and cry, and my own tears flowed down my cheeks. My protective instincts were to pull her form the flood of sub-zero water, and hold her close to my body to warm her. I knew I had to continue to get her fever back down.

I watched as every part of her body turned to a cold, dark blue, bordering on a purplish black. I sobbed uncompromisingly and could not hold her in the freezing water any longer. I grabbed a towel as I pulled her from the tub, wrapping her naked body and drawing her in close to my chest. I rubbed her arms to warm her, and return her to a flush, warm pink, again.

The nurse found me sobbing uncontrollably, attempting to warm my daughter, as my tears fell across her little face. She reached over and pulled her from my arms.

She said, "No honey, you don't want to do this. I know how hard it is, but we want to cool her to bring her fever down. "I'm sorry you had to do this," she said, laying Jeni-lee back into her crib, wearing only a loosely fitted diaper.

The weekend passed without a confirmed diagnosis. Dr. Lennox returned as scheduled and said her fever was under control and he still detected a croup sound in her lungs.

"I think your daughter is suffering from asthma," he said, revealing his diagnosis to me.

"Asthma? ASTHMA? I yelled a second time. A rage came over me, a righteous anger that said this was a lie of the devil.

I stepped forward, into Dr. Lennox's personal space, stared him in the eye, and firmly said aloud, "I rebuke you devil! You're a liar and I cast down every evil lie spoken over my daughter. SHE DOES NOT HAVE ASTHMA IN JESUS NAME!"

Dr. Lennox took a step back away from me with a stunned expression. He paused silently for a moment before softly whispering, "I'll look at some more tests and let you know what I find out," he said averting his eyes from mine.

I turned back toward Michael and said, "It doesn't matter what they find now! My daughter is healed in JESUS name! The devil is a liar and I know he comes to steal, kill and destroy and he is not getting my daughter in Jesus name. The victory is mine," I declared aloud

Michael took me into his arms and held me until I calmed down.

We returned to Jeni-lee's room and quietly prayed.

The nurse came in and said that her fever had broken and we raced for the victory line that was right in front of us. We had won!

Michael returned home, and I slept in two hour periodicals as the nurses came in and out through the night.

It was a new morning and Dr. Lennox returned to tell me the tests revealed pneumonia and febrile seizures. "She is doing very well right now and I will be sending her home with you this morning," he said, smiling. "She will be prone to febrile seizures in the future, so watch her closely."

"Should you have any complications, call my office or bring her back to ER immediately. I assure you, she is fine now," he confirmed.

I smiled and we immediately scooped up our daughter and returned home, thanking God for the miracles in our life.

Chapter 7
MINISTRY

We settled back into our everyday routines while Michael's alcohol driven benders became more frequent.

In most instances, he would vanish, ranging from overnight, to sometimes, as long as two weeks. It seems he was away, more than he was home these days. He had been slowly returning to his old self, before salvation. Often times, I wondered if he loved us at all. He wouldn't return home until he tired of the bars, the constant partying, and the women, whom he conned into supplying his addictions. When he did return home, the fights exploded with greater intensity, each time. It seemed I couldn't make him stop drinking, but I couldn't give up on him, or stop trying.

I continued to speak diligent morning prayers, begging God to make Michael stop drinking. I wondered if it were my lack of faith, or if sobriety for him, was even possible.

Jeni-lee was four months old now. I made her a pallet on the floor, and laid her on her belly, hoping she would crawl to her toys that I had strategically placed around her. Michael and I were studying our bibles when I looked over to see if she was trying to crawl. She had rolled over to her back where she lay, very still and quiet. I moved toward her to see her eyes drooping, with a blank stare. She was congested and her breathing became shallow. I took her temperature and it read 101 F.

I anxiously lifted her into my arms, and yelled for Michael. "We have to take her back to ER right now! I think she is starting to seizure again," I said running for the car.

Dr. Lennox met us at the ER and treated her with antibiotics in an I.V and sent us home with a Tylenol prescription. I stayed up with her most of the night, fearing a repeat episode of febrile seizures.

Over the course of the next year, we were in and out of the ER at least twice a month. Occasionally, Jeni-lee was hospitalized and other times she was sent home with antibiotics and Tylenol. I was puzzled, wondering what was causing her constant illness. I fed her fresh, organic vegetables from my garden, hoping it would help her to stay healthy, but to no avail.

Through it all, the Lord pricked Michael's heart with the conviction of us living together, unmarried, and in sin. We sat down to lunch and he told me that Jesus was telling him to marry me right away.

"We've been living together for years now, maybe it's time we set thing right, Judith. I just want us to be a real family in the eyes of God," he said with conviction.

"Yes," I said elated. God has been convicting my heart since I was pregnant with Jeni-lee," I said.

We set a date in Late September and decided to have a small ceremony in our home, only inviting John and Joyce as witnesses, and of course, our parents.

Michael had found a new Christian friend, named Randy. They spent a lot of time together and Randy took it upon himself to begin counseling Michael. He shared the word of God with Michael, brother to brother, hoping to help him find deliverance from his addictions.

Randy quickly became Michael's brother and confidant. He had confided, not only his addictions and his conviction to marry me, but he also confided our personal struggles in our relationship with Randy.

It was a September afternoon, and a cool breeze swept through the house. I had finished my chores and was playing with the children, when Michael and Randy strolled through the front door.

I offered Randy a seat and a glass of iced tea.

Michael interrupted and said, "Judith, we would like to talk to you for a few minutes. Will you join us, and listen carefully to something we would like to share with you?"

"Okay," I said puzzled at his odd request. I sent the boys off to play and joined them in the living room.

Randy shared with me their discussion about Michael's problems, and the causes therein, according to the word of God.

"It's you, Judith. You are a witch, practicing in witchcraft," Randy's mind boggling accusation rang loudly in my ears. "You need to repent, renounce and break off the witchcraft, so Michael can begin to heal. Only then, can you be a family, centered in Christ. If you refuse, Michael cannot marry you," he solemnly announced.

I froze, stunned by his words. After a moment, I sprung defensively to my feet yelling, "What? What are you talking about? You're crazy!" I stared at him, baffled by his accusation. I was surprised that Michael would believe any of this. I glanced back and forth between Michael and Randy, waiting for Michael to speak up, in my defense.

Michael immediately raised his hand, as if to defend Randy's accusation and tell me to be quiet.

I stepped back and shouted, "I am not a witch! How dare you! You two have no idea what you're talking about! Really? Do you think I cast spells over Michael to make him drink? You are nuts! I am not a witch," I decreed in sheer exasperation at this horrific accusation.

"That's it! Get out of my house, Randy," I said pointing my finger at Randy. I slowly stepped in toward Randy, in a threatening manner and ordered, "Get Out!"

Michael jumped between us, calmly suggesting that Randy leave, so he could speak with me alone.

"Let's sit down and talk about this, Judith," Michael coolly suggested.

I continued to pace in anger and asked, "What is wrong with you, Michael? You know I'm not a witch. Oh my God, why are you listening to this man? He is obviously a sick and disturbed man," I blurted in disgust.

"Listen to me! He doesn't mean that kind of witch," Michael articulated, unconvincingly.

"Well, what other kind of witch is there, Michael?" I yelled, throwing my hands into the air.

"Judith, will you calm down and listen? He means a spiritual witch. The kind of witch that controls others, manipulating them," Michael argued.

You're crazy! In fact, you're both crazy! Oh my God, I am not going to have this stupid, ridiculous conversation with you, and furthermore, don't ever bring that man back into my house again, or so help me, Michael, you will regret it! How's that for control?" I roared, spewing my venom all over him. I walked away to prevent the argument from escalating into a physical confrontation.

We moved forward, having bible studies and praying for his sobriety. One afternoon he went off to meet with his new and trusted friend, Randy. I was uncomfortable with their friendship, but I knew Randy would not encourage him to go out drinking.

Michael soon returned home, inviting me to have another conversation with him.

He described a Christian Rehabilitation Ranch, located in the mountains that set behind us, near Idyllwild. Michael said that he and Randy had agreed, if I were not willing to admit that I was a witch and get help, it would be best if he left me and stayed at the Ranch. He said he would agree to child visitations once he was released from the Ranch.

Shocked and bewildered, I replied, "Randy said for you to leave me? I don't believe this! You said it was God's will for us to get married. What happened? Randy said you should leave me, so you listen to him, instead of God?"

"I just can't figure you out?" I said, astonished. "What about our children? You're going to just abandon us all together because I won't admit to being a witch?" I said appalled at his threat.

"You don't understand, this is what God wants me to do first. I have to find sobriety, deliverance, and healing, and you have to get delivered before we can get married. Perhaps we can discuss reconciliation after I graduate the ranch, that is, if you are willing to make changes as well, and if its God's will," he said attempting to convince me that I was the problem.

"Randy is going to the Ranch with me. His wife understands, why can't you, Judith? For the first 30 days, I can't have any outside contact, but here is the number you can reach me at, after the 30 days have passed," he said, laying the written phone number on the coffee table.

Michael went into the bedroom to pack as I paced, incensed at his words.

"Fine, but if you go this time, we are through. I am finished with all this nonsense. Don't bother calling me, in fact, don't ever call me again. I hate you! Just get out and stay out," I yelled.

Randy parked in front of our gate and I watched as Michael got into the car and drove away.

Confused and not knowing exactly how I should feel, I had a sudden urge to draw a picture of a house on construction paper. I cut out a large heart, and cut the heart in two, as if to resemble a broken heart. I glued it in the center of the house, with Michael on one side, and the children and I on the other side, because were a family divided. I took a string of yarn, anointed it, and tied it over the house, hanging the entire sheet on my bedroom wall. I prayed, if it be thy will, Lord heal my home, allowing us to reconcile and marry. I walked away still swearing off any relationship with Michael, ever again.

It had been six weeks since Michael left. Our phone service had been disconnected and I received messages on my mother's phone. My youngest brother, Kelly, delivered a message, telling me Michael had called and requested that I call him back.

I returned his call the next day. Michael said he had to leave the Ranch immediately. He explained that it turned out to be a cult. He wasn't allowed to speak for very long, so he quickly asked if I would borrow my mother's car and come to pick him up that evening. He whispered, not wanting to be heard by others. He told me he would have to sneak out of the ranch, and described a tree located at the property line where he would meet me at 10:00 p.m.

After Michael returned home, he told me about the mayhem at the Ranch, and we moved on in an attempt to reconcile our separation, and marital status. He apologized, asking if we could marry as soon as possible.

We set the date for January 12, 1984. I counted our pennies, and planned our wedding as inexpensively as possible.

Our wedding day had arrived. I wore a silver dress with a silvery, blue bridal bouquet. Our friends, John and Joyce attended, bringing with them some punch and a beautiful wedding cake. Both our parents, along with Pastor Browning and his wife, Mary Nell attended. We were quietly married in our home, just as we had planned. Finally, after nine long years, we were a family, in right standing before God, and we were a joyfully, blessed family indeed.

The months passed and we continued to take Jeni-lee to visit the ER. I had read an article about the glue in pressed board, emitting toxins into the air when exposed to heat. Our mobile home was made from pressed board. I suggested to Michael that we move into a house, to see if it would make a difference in her health.

We relocated to our new home, just a few blocks away. It needed some minor repairs and we set out to dig up the leach lines and make repairs to the house. Once we were settled, we filled the wooden storage shed in the back yard, with donations for the needy. We stored food, clothing, toiletries and bibles. Before we knew it, our ministry was taking off. Our storage shed was quickly diminishing as we donated to the needy, and replenished again, by God through word of mouth.

A displaced couple with two small children, fell on hard times, and came to church, asking for help. We drove to the motel where they stayed, introduced ourselves, and offered to help.

We became fast friends, inviting them to our home for a weekly bible study together, adopting them as our new family in Christ Jesus.

One afternoon, Michael ran to the market for some milk, while I went to the kitchen to work on my award winning chili.

Michael returned and said, "I hope you don't mind, but I brought a couple of homeless men back to join us for dinner. It was just amazing, Judith! I saw them jump off the train, when I felt the Lord instructing me to bring them home and minister to them. I hope it's okay with you," he said.

"Of course it's okay. Where are they?"

"They're outside. They smell really bad and refused to come in. I told them they can't bring their wine inside. I thought they could maybe use the bathroom to clean up," he hinted.

"I'll take care of this," I said stubbornly and walked out to introduce myself. They called themselves, lil Mac, and big Mac. Lil Mac, was about 5' 7" and maybe 150 lbs. He was a friendly, outgoing little man, with no teeth and badly bruised over his entire body. Big Mac stood about 6' 4", and around 230 lbs. He was very introvert, skeptical and a very distrusting fellow.

I demanded they both come into the house and make full use of the shower. I have clean clothes and toiletries for you. Afterwards, we will have dinner and then we will sit and visit awhile," I said, inviting them.

I was surprised when they went into the bathroom together. Michael explained that they didn't trust us. They were hobo's and closer than brothers.

After showering, both men returned to the living room. Michael witnessed to the downtrodden, whimsical men, both called Mac. They listened intently and lil Mac asked questions about salvation, and I listened as Michael answered him.

Suddenly, Jeni-lee leapt into lil Mac's lap, reaching up to stroke the side of his face and smiled, looking intently into his eyes before sliding back off of his lap and running off again to play.

Lil Mac covered his face and began to cry.

"Why are you crying, lil Mac?" I asked, concerned.

Lil Mac opened up, and told us his story. He had been living in Florida with his wife and children. His wife divorced him and he became an alcoholic, eventually leading him to homelessness. He tried to remain a part of his children's and grandchildren's lives, but was told to stay away and never come near his grandchildren again. He told us that he was amazed that we allowed Jeni-lee to sit in his lap and love on him. He sobbed, "I am just a filthy, worthless old man, and I can't believe there are still people like you and your family, left in this world."

"Yes, I want to accept Jesus into my heart as my Lord and Savior, but first, there is something I have to do," he exclaimed, walking toward the front door.

"C'mon Mac," he said bolting out the front door. We watched in surprise as they emptied their 2 liter coke bottles that had been filled with wine, into the dirt.

Michael and I looked at each other, and just smiled.

"You don't have to do that," Michael said.

"I want to," lil Mac said, grinning. His face lit with joy.

We watched as they washed out their bottles with dish soap and filled them with fresh water, to travel with. They returned inside to say the sinner's prayer with us, receiving Jesus as their personal Savior.

I packed each of them, a duffle bag filled with a bible, a change of clothes and some snacks.

Lil Mac stood upright and said, "We gotta get going now. We are going to stand at the freeway onramp, all cleaned up, and hitch a ride back to Florida. I'm going home to see my children and grandchildren. I want them to see the new creation I am, because Jesus died for me," he proclaimed. "I want my family back and I believe Jesus will do it for me. I swear, I will never drink again."

Michael drove them to the I-10 freeway onramp after we prayed again and said our good byes.

Throughout the coming weeks the Lord continued to send frightened saints, and lost sinners, some to our door, and some by telephone. Distressed and abused women in relationships with men having addictions, began to seek me out. We had become very busy with the Lord's work.

Meanwhile, Jeni-lee was perpetually sick. The ER trips and occasional hospital stays continued.

Michael researched possible solutions for her constant illnesses. He searched the bible as well as other literature for answers. After a time, he diagnosed Jeni-lee as suffering from a spirit of rejection, based on my not wanting another child during my pregnancy with her.

He explained, in essence, Jeni-lee subconsciously felt rejected, unwanted, undesired, unloved and believed she had no right to life. Therefore, her medical episodes were a form of suicide. She had been experiencing this from birth. He explained that I needed to repent for not wanting another child, or the pregnancy, before God could heal her. After I had done this, we would take turns, whispering affirmations of her right to life, freedom, salvation, success, education, and happiness into her ear, as she fell asleep.

Michael was without a doubt, convincingly persuasive in his diagnosis and argument for Jen-lee's healing. I realized that we are not changed from the outside, but from the inside out. We whispered affirmations and observed an immediate difference. There were no more ER trips or hospital stays.

Jeni-lee's third birthday was approaching quickly. We went to see Kris and Andy on our way to the market. We extended an invitation to them for Jeni-lee's upcoming birthday party. They accepted and before leaving, we prayed for Andy, who had been suffering with severe depression.

We drove into the Alpha Beta parking lot slowly, searching for a parking space. Immediately, we observed an anomalous sight. A two man tent, was pitched next to a parked car in the middle of the parking lot. In front of the tent were two camping chairs, where a man and a woman sat, holding a sign that read, "PLEASE HELP!"

We finished our shopping and loaded our trunk with groceries. When we had finished, we walked over to greet the young couple sitting in their camping chairs. They introduced themselves as Brian and Tawana. They had been living together and they both had lost their jobs, along with everything else except for their car and the few items that we saw in front of us.

"We are desperate and decided to plant ourselves in the middle of the parking lot, hoping someone would offer us a chance," Brian confessed.

Michael offered Brian and Tawana, a three month stay in Jeni-lee's bedroom and help finding work, on the condition that they clean up after themselves and buy their own food. They followed us home and Michael immediately ministered the word of God to them.

I spoke with my mother, who offered them both employment at the Wheel Inn Truck Stop, where she worked as a manager.

We watched as our ministry grew. We had regular bible studies, donations for the needy, deliverance ministry, and evangelized the public whenever we went to town.

Michael continued his bouts and disappointments with his addictions.

I sat under an open window, on a cool, partly cloudy, Thursday afternoon. Michael would be leaving for L.A. to work a temporary construction job for two weeks. I suspected he had been drinking the last couple of weeks and had an uneasy feeling in the pit of my stomach.

Suddenly, I heard that still small voice, once again. "Go to your mother." I wondered if it were me or the Lord. Once more, I heard the gentle voice, "Go to your mother, now."

I parked in front of my mother's gate and saw George sitting in his usual spot in his garage. I entered into the house, breathing in the fresh brewed aroma of coffee.

I looked over to see my mother's head laying on her arms across the top of the table, with her head bobbing up and down as she sobbed. I had only seen her cry three times in my life, and wondered what had happened to make her cry so hard.

I ran to ask her what happened. She drew in several long desperate, gasps of air, attempting to speak.

"Daryl is going to die today, I just know it," she said, fighting to form her words through her gasps for air.

Aghast at her remark, I said, "Daryl is at work and he's fine."

"He came home for lunch and I begged him not to go back," she moaned weary from her tears. "He's going to die on that motorcycle today, I just know it. I never should have co-signed for him to get that bike," she said pounding her fist against the table.

Bewildered and taken aback by her words, I reached out to comfort her. "No, mom, Daryl is okay. I know he is okay. I'll sit with you until he returns, then you'll see for yourself.

Nearly two hours had passed and I was unable to console her. "Look mom, it's nearly time for Daryl to come home," I said. I cupped her hands into mine when I heard someone pull up in front of the house.

To my chagrin, it wasn't Daryl, but a Riverside County sheriff. The sheriff stepped out of his car and yelled to George in the garage, Daryl? I was horrified at realizing my mother's fears had just become a reality.

"Oh my God, it's not Daryl, it's the sheriff, I said as I went to the door.

I ran to the sheriff who stood with his arm resting over the top of the gate. George hollered, "What about Daryl?"

"Daryl has been in an accident. He was taken to Desert Regional Hospital," he reported.

"Is he okay," I asked

"I can't say," the sheriff responded uncomfortably.

"I ran back inside to find my mother on the floor, wailing like a wounded animal, and pounding her fists, as she gasped for enough oxygen to sing her words, "No, no, no, no!

I reached down, attempting to pull her to her feet and told her Daryl had been in an accident. We needed to drive to the hospital, more than twenty miles away. I laid her twisted body into the recliner as she screamed hysterically, "He's dead!"

I ran back outside to the sheriff and asked, "Is my brother still alive?"

The sheriff looked at me reluctantly, and said, "I don't have that information."

I positioned my stance as I pointed my finger behind me toward the front door, and asked again, "Is my brother still alive? My mother is in hysterics and collapsed on the floor. She is crying hysterically, "He is dead," over and over, again and I have to tell her something. So, I ask you again, Sir, is my brother still alive?"

The Sheriff hesitated and his expression turned to sincere compassion, as he told me he didn't know if Daryl was still alive or not. "He was still alive when I left him at the accident site. His injuries are very serious. If I were you, I wouldn't waste any time taking your mother to the hospital," he said, averting his eyes from mine.

I ran back inside to find my mother on the phone, incoherently mumbling the words, "Daryl is dead." I pried the phone from her fingers to hear Trishly's panicked voice, "What's going on?"

I told her what I knew and asked her to meet us at the Hospital Trauma Unit.

I threw my arms around my mother's weak, limp body and guided her to the nurse's window, where we inquired about Daryl's condition. He was still alive but had sustained serious head injury. The nurse took my mother to the back to see him, while I immediately called Michael from the hospital to let him know I would not be home any time soon. He agreed to wait a couple of days before going to L.A. for his temporary job assignment.

Daryl's recovery was now a waiting game. My mother returned to the waiting room and I watched as the tears steadily streamed over her cheeks. She stood there in a state of shock, after seeing Daryl.

Suddenly, she turned, and positioned herself to attack and defend. With her fists swinging wildly, she violently beat the wall, kicking her feet, and screaming, "No, no, no.

"With a firm and strong voice, she yelled, "I will fight You, God, or whoever you are. Do you hear me? I won't let You have my son, You won't take him from me, because I won't let You! I'll fight You, do You hear me, I'll fight You?"

I listened as the nurse called security for a hysterical woman in the waiting room. Fearful for my mother, I pulled her into me, holding her close against my body, and wrapping my arms around her. I whispered, "Put your arms around me, mom, and squeeze. Squeeze tight and hold on, he will be okay." She held tight, squeezing the breath from me, and she suddenly pulled away and said, "I'm okay now, with her fists still clenched in front of her.

Daryl, was in an induced coma for his own protection. The next day, they took him in for brain surgery, and we waited.

Saturday evening the doctor came in to tell us that Daryl was improving, and we should all go home, promising to call if there were any change.

I returned home, exhausted after three days in a waiting room. I showered and shared the story of praying the sinner's prayer with Daryl and that I knew, that I knew, in my heart that even if Daryl died, God would raise him back to life. Michael reminded me that he would be leaving in the morning for L.A.

Morning came and I was cleaning up after breakfast when the phone rang. It was George.

"Yeah, the hospital called and they said Daryl is dying. You better get here now."

Overwhelmed by his shocking words, I wept. I wiped my eyes and returned to the hospital.

My family gathered at the ICU waiting room, where we met the doctor.

"We are doing everything humanly possible," the doctor told us. His ceratoid artery has ruptured, stopping all blood flow to the brain. He is currently sustained by life support. Does anyone know if Daryl left directives concerning life support? You will have to make the decision, whether or not to keep him life support, soon."

We all agreed that Daryl had voiced that he didn't want to live on life support.

I went to the chapel to pray. It was time for that miracle. My faith was certain at this point. I returned to ICU waiting, to rejoin my parents, and wait for our miracle.

I sat beside my mother, holding my bible and praying as I gazed upward to the corner of the corridor, across from me. I witnessed something manifest and hover in that corner. It was transparent, without form or color, but resembled the shape of a man. My awareness heightened as I watched the entity begin to move slowly toward me. I experienced a sudden awareness that if this entity touched me, my brother would die, never to return. I wanted to get up and run, but my body froze, rendering me unable to move. Feeling threatened by the possibility of Daryl's death being permanent, I threw my legs into the air, screaming, "No, no, no," in an attempt to block this entity from ever touching me. I abruptly felt the weight of the entity lie across my body, pressing in on me, and I knew my brother wasn't coming back.

My mother grabbed my arm and squeezed, as she gazed at me questionably. Suddenly, I remembered the prophetic words spoken that day in church, almost three years ago. "Do not fear for this young man, for I have claimed him as my own dear son, and he will soon be with me." I wept, realizing that this was a literal prophecy.

The doctor returned to tell us that it was only a matter of time before his heart and lungs gave out under the life support. It was time to make that decision.

"Have you made a decision?" The doctor calmly asked.

"Yes," my mother replied, mustering every ounce of courage and strength, for that moment. We have decided to remove him from life support, but I will be in the room beside him, holding him in my arms when you turn it off. My son came into this world through my body, and he will leave this world through my body," she said in fragmented, broken words, as her tears flooded her beautifully set cheek bones, and her body trembled.

The doctor agreed to her terms and set a time later that morning to turn off the machines.

"You understand it could take several minutes, even up to an hour for his body to completely shut down, don't you?" The doctor asked.

"I don't care! I will hold him in my arms until the last beat of his heart," my mother cried.

I left the hospital that Monday afternoon. The clouds hung low in the valley, and there was a cool, light rain, misting over my face as I walked through the parking lot. My hot, steamy tears were hidden by the small rain drops that pelted across my face. There was a vast emptiness in my belly, and a crater sized hole in my heart, silencing my every thought and emotion, leaving me numb. I was leaving the hospital that day with one less family member to love, to spend holidays with, to grow old with, and to share my memories with.

I returned home to find that Michael had left for L.A., leaving the children with Brian and Tawana until I returned home.

I sent my children off to play, while I drowned myself in my sorrows and self-pity, realizing I would never see or speak to my little brother again. I questioned his salvation and reminded Jesus that it wasn't too late, He could still raise him from the dead. Confusion settled in, and I wondered why God would hurt me like this.

I awoke to the sound of caterwauling as the kids fought over the cereal. I fed them, cleaned up after them, and sent the boys outside to play while Jeni-lee went into her room to play with her Barbie's.

Brian and Tawana awoke to join me for coffee and tea later that morning, offering their sympathies. They poured a second cup and returned to their room, together.

From the silence, I heard an alarmingly, piercing scream, impaling my ears, causing me to leap to my feet. Jeni-lee ran toward me, leapt onto my legs and began her ascent to the very top of my head, as though I were a tree.

She didn't stop until she sat on the top of my head, holding on to my hair, and screaming hysterically.

Brian and Tawana bolted from their room to see what the commotion was all about, and I struggled to remove Jeni-lee from the top of my head. She fought me, kicking and screaming so hard, Tawana had to help remove, and untangle her from my hair. I held her in my arms, asking her what had happened.

She relentlessly continued to scream a shrill, high pitched, assaulting scream. I attempted to set her on the floor and she fought to hang on to me. I forced her to the floor as she screamed, unyieldingly, and her tiny hands fought to hold something back away from her legs. She cowered as if to move away from some invisible attacker.

My eyes opened wide and my jaw dropped in disbelief. I saw large, human like, bite marks appear on her little legs, but there was nothing there to bite her.

"Oh my God! Do you see that?" Tawana shrieked, pointing at Jeni-lee's legs.

We looked on as more bite marks embedded deeply into her flesh, breaking the skin but not quite deep enough to draw blood. They were painful and Jeni-lee continued to scream.

I lifted her into my protective arms, realizing this was a demonic attack.

Brian and Tawana were struck with fear. Perturbed in the unbelief of their hearts, Brian said, "This is too weird for us. I'm sorry Judith, but we have to leave. We'll be back for our things later and drove away a moment later.

Several minutes later, Brian and Tawana returned. "Judith, you won't believe what happened a couple of miles from here. We were leaving Cabazon, minding our own business, and out of nowhere, this ghostly looking thing circled around our car, surrounding us. We got so scared! We didn't know what to do, so we came back here. This is scary! What should we do?" Brian asked, confused and frightened.

"Just keep praying while I make some phone calls for help," I told him. After calling every known resource for prayer, I decided it was time to call Michael home.

I called the emergency number he had left me, and asked to speak to Michael. I explained our dire situation and begged him to return home as soon as possible. I could almost smell the alcohol on his breath through the phone, as he slurred his words. Michael refused my urgent request, using our need for finances as his reasoning. I argued with him, when suddenly, Tawana snatched the receiver from my hand.

"You need to come back home immediately," she firmly spoke into the receiver. "Your wife and children need you here. Your brother in law is dead, your daughter is hysterical, and your wife is on the verge of collapsing! What kind of father and husband are you, anyway? You dare to call yourself a Christian man," she charged.

After a moment of silence, she hung up the receiver and said, "Okay, Michael will be home in the morning."

Morning came and Jeni-lee had laid on top of me, clinging tightly to my neck through the night. Michael returned home shortly after we woke up. When Jeni-lee saw him, she stretched out her arms and leapt onto him like a wild cat.

Michael called an immediate household meeting. We prayed in agreement, asking the Lord to show us where the evil was coming from. He questioned each of us, asking if we had brought anything new into the home. He asked if I had brought any memorabilia home belonging to Daryl, or any keepsakes.

"No, I only brought my purse home," I said irritated with his questioning.

After searching the house and continual prayer, Michael turned toward Brian and said, "It's you! What is in your pockets? We have searched everything. It must be on your person," he said, pushing Brian. "Empty your pockets on the table," Michael insisted.

Annoyed at Michael's accusation, Brian emptied his right, front pocket, spilling his change onto the table. Then he removed his keys from his left front pocket, tossing them on to the table.

"There it is, Michael said, reaching over to lift Brian's keys.

"They are just keys," Brian exclaimed.

"It's your key ring. This is a pentagram! You are carrying this pentagram on your key ring and it's a talisman or amulet. Why?" Michael interrogated.

"I bought it because I thought it was cool, and the man said it would bring me good luck," Brian said defensively. "I didn't know it represented anything evil."

"It is used in witchcraft to conjure up evil spirits. It is a portal, or door way to an evil, spiritual realm. When you brought this into my house, you opened the door for evil to enter legally, and harm my family," Michael said, educating Brian. "Now take it off my property. You may not keep it in your room or in your car while it sits on my property," Michael warned.

We prayed over Jeni-lee, and our home, anointing each room with oil and she returned to the peaceful, joy filled little girl she was before all of this.

Brian and Tawana married each other, and had saved enough money to get their own home and move away.

Michael, finally landed a dream job, making five times the current minimum wage he had been earning. He drove for a linen delivery service. After a week and a half, he was fired for drinking and driving on the job.

I desperately sought peace over my brother's death and there seemed to be none. I questioned his salvation and had repetitive nightmares. Michael's drinking was raging out of control and I was constantly on edge. Torment began to whittle away at my spirit, little by little.

I found liquor bottles hidden behind the toilet, under the mattress and in a wood pile in the back yard. Michael's drinking was raging out of control once more. One morning, I awoke to the quiet emptiness of my bed. He had left for another bender in the night, as I slept. The children and I spent the day together, played, did chores and watched some television and the day passed slowly.

Evening came and I put the kids to bed. Jeni-lee was afraid to sleep in her room alone, and fell asleep on the love seat, near me.

I knelt to my knees beside the sofa and began to pray, beseeching God for Michael's sobriety. The hours passed as I cried, and sobbed in my aloneness, struggles and fears. My misery manifested into a pool of salty tears and snot, manifesting into grief, fear and helplessness. I bargained, promised and plead with God into the wee morning hours, asking Him to return my husband to me, sober and safe.

I jumped as Jeni-lee pulled herself to her feet over the back of the sofa, looked out the window and said, "He's coming. Daddy is coming around the mountain." As quickly as she had leapt to her feet, she laid down, without ever awakening or reaching consciousness.

Was God speaking through her? If he were coming around the mountain, that means he is about fifteen minutes away. I ran to the bathroom to wash my face and hide my tears. Returning to the sofa, I continued to pray.

Fifteen minutes had passed, and it was now 3:00 a.m. The phone rang, startling me to my feet. It was Michael, calling from the Cabazon Country Market, asking if he could come home.

"Yes, we need for you to come home, please come home," I cried.

I immediately praised God for this wonderful miracle in my life.

Michael walked in, and with crimson red, tear filled eyes, I fell into his arms and kissed him.

He shared with me how this miracle had happened. He was sitting in a bar, drinking, when a strange man approached him and shared Jesus, convincing him to return home to his family.

In turn, I shared with him about Jeni-lee's prophetic words, and we rejoiced in the love and amazing grace of our Lord and Savior, Jesus Christ.

Chapter 8
A LIFE OF Chaos

Finally, I received a job offer in Palm Springs, paying me twice what minimum wage was paying, plus tips. I leapt at the opportunity and loved my new job.

I rode to work with my younger sister, who was also employed there while I prayed for a new car. We worked the swing shift, from two to ten in the evenings and every weekend. My children were usually asleep when I returned home, and at school when I awoke in the morning.

Before long, God answered my prayer and we were gifted a nearly new, Dodge colt, station wagon. Once I had transportation, my employer required a lot of overtime from me, decreasing the time I was able to spend with my family.

With spring approaching, the restaurant slowed and the manager released me early, to spend some much needed time with my family.

I returned home to find Jimmy and Jeffrey locked out of the house, playing in the front yard. When I asked where Michael was, Jimmy said, "Dad took Jeni-lee and went to the store a long time ago.

I put the boys in the car and drove out in search of Michael and Jeni-lee.

I was nearing the wash when I spotted him weaving as he drove toward home. I stopped him, removed Jeni-lee from the car and when he refused to ride with me, I said I'd follow him home.

Michael staggered into the living room, surprised by my early return. I railed against him for endangering our children's lives, as well as his own, and he profusely apologized. He realized what he had done and promised to never let it happen again.

I continued to work the long grueling days of constant overtime, for a straight twenty four days, with no time off. I hadn't seen my children for nearly a month, and was sorely missing them. I got up early one morning, sent the kids off to school, allowing Michael to sleep in, and called the restaurant to tell them I wouldn't be in today.

I spent the day with my daughter and my husband. Jimmy and Jeffrey were excited, to find me home when they returned from school. We spent the afternoon playing games and watching television.

After dinner, the boys went in to share a bath together. I looked down the hallway, from the end of the sofa, where I sat watching the boys run into the bathroom.

Jimmy darted from the bathroom to return to his room to get a toy that he had forgotten. Wearing only his white briefs, I spotted large patches of dirt on his back as he returned to the bathroom with his toy.

I went to the bathroom to investigate, wondering how he had gotten so dirty. He hadn't been outside, except at school. He grabbed the shower curtain and wrapped it around his body when I entered, hiding his nakedness.

"Jimmy, what is on your back? Turn around so I can see. How did you get dirt on your back?" I asked him.

"No mommy, It's okay. I'll wash my back," his lip quivered and he seemed to be frightened.

"You don't have to be embarrassed. I won't look at you, Jimmy. I just want to see your back," I said, reaching for his shoulder to turn him around.

He cried aloud, "I'm bad mommy! It's okay, because I am bad and I deserved it. I was a bad boy. Please don't be mad, mommy!"

Looking over his back, I was fixed in disbelief. Taken aback by the evidence in front of me, I realized it wasn't dirt at all, it was black and blue bruising from his shoulders to his knees.

"Who did this to you, Jimmy?" I asked him, stunned by the sight of his backside. "Who? Tell me who did this to you? Was it papa? Was it someone at school? Tell me, Jimmy, who did it?" I asked, demanding an answer.

"No mommy, I was very bad and I deserved it. I can't tell you, mommy, please," he said, refusing to divulge the name of the person, who had done this atrocious thing.

I left the boys to finish their bath and told Michael what I had found. "I can't imagine who could have done such a thing," I told him.

"Maybe he fell," Michael said, unconcerned. "He's always playing rough," he suggested.

After seeing the bruises for himself, Michael agreed, this was no fall, or accident.

The following morning, I kept the boys home from school, and suggested we call the police.

"I want to find out who did this first, before we tell anyone," Michael said, as he warned me that the authorities may try to take our children from us.

Determined to find out who had done this to my son, I took Jimmy aside after breakfast and held him in my arms, confirming to him that he was a good boy, and I loved him very much. I told him he didn't deserve to be hit by anyone. I promised to protect him, and never allow anyone to do this to him again, no matter who it was. I promised him, I wouldn't get angry, and I would listen to him. "Who was it, Jimmy?" I asked again.

After a moment of silent apprehension, Jimmy revealed, "It was daddy. I was very bad and he got really mad. I deserved it and I promise to be a good boy from now on, mommy," Jimmy said crying, as he wiped his eyes.

"Dad? Daddy did this to you? Tell me what he did, Jimmy."

"Daddy was drinking and he wasn't supposed to. I told him not to drink and made him mad. He sent all of us to our room. He sat Jeffrey and Jeni-lee down by the wall and made me take off my pants and my shirt. Then he made me spread my legs and grab the top bunk bed with my arms spread. He said he was going to whip me with my hot wheel track, thirty three times, one stripe for every year that Jesus lived. He whipped me and made me count each one out loud. He stopped when I said thirty three. Then he said, if we told anyone, he would do the same thing to Jeffrey and Jeni-lee. Please mommy, don't be mad," Jimmy detailed the events to me, with a broken spirit.

I pulled him in close to me and held him, promising him that I would never let anyone hurt him again.

I took the children to Jeni-lee's bedroom and locked them in, while I confronted Michael.

"GET OUT," I roared as a lioness, protecting her cubs. I reached for a butcher knife to keep him away from me and screamed, "You did this to Jimmy!"

He immediately shielded himself by blaming me, "Your never home and I felt trapped. I am trying to change," he said, pleading for another chance.

When I refused to negotiate, he hollered, "No, I'm not leaving without my share of the money and the car," he argued.

"You're not getting anything," I declared! I will call the police and I'll call your dad to settle our disagreement about the car. I have a job and am supporting our children. You, on the other hand, want to get drunk and sleep in the car."

I called his father immediately. He agreed that he had gifted us both with the car, but under the circumstances, I should keep the car to continue to support our children. I rethought the idea of calling the police, for fear that CPS would take my children for failing to protect, while I worked, unaware of what was going on in my own home.

Michael soon left our home and disappeared.

Unable to obtain a babysitter for the night time hours I was required to work, I lost my job and was forced to apply for welfare benefits.

The requests for prayer from women whose husbands were drinking, using drugs, and neglecting their children, or abusing them, began to pour in.

Kris called to request prayer for Andy, who was at an all-time low in his depression. My mother asked me to help her manage her household, the neighbors needed prayer, my sister was crushed by her boyfriend's lack of desire to marry her, nightmares of Daryl's death haunted me, and the problems kept right on pouring in. I was struggling to keep my head just barely above water, drowning in my multiple sorrows and losses.

Feeling overwhelmed with sadness and depression, but no time to wallow in it, I sat on the edge of my bed to pray. My tears flowed endlessly.

I closed my eyes and questioned God about Daryl's death, the demonic attack against my daughter, the beating of my son by his dad, our separation, the loss of my job and the list went on. These were not small things and I didn't understand why God was not protecting me. "Why, God? Why?" I cried aloud.

I listened to the water trickle and there was a song in the breeze, as I breathed in the most unbelievable air. Suddenly, the atmosphere had changed. I opened my eyes to see an incredible light, filling the environment that surrounded me. The open skies over me were endless and the light was alive and breathed, drawing me in. There was a stream below the grass covered knoll where I sat, surrounded by trees and beautiful flowers. There were the most unspeakable, vibrant colors I had never encountered. The pulsating flowers, majestic trees, and every blade of grass, swayed in rhythm to the song in the breeze that brushed across my cheek. Everything was so alive, so unspeakably beautiful. The whole of everything had breath and breathed in a new, perfect life. A perfect, faultless peace surrounded and engulfed me, when suddenly, I heard a voice. I turned to look toward the voice and saw my little brother, Daryl. He was sitting on the knoll beside me and he was filled with an indescribable contentment, peace, and joy. There was a renewed strength and confidence inhabiting his entire existence. "Daryl," I cried…..

"Judith, why do you cry for me? Don't you understand, even if I could, I don't want to return to that life! Look around you. Why would I want to leave? I love you, Judith. Do not cry for me! Tell mom, I am sorry I hurt her. Tell her, I love her," he boldly declared.

173

I opened my eyes to find myself sitting in the darkness of my bedroom, on the edge of my bed. "What happened? It was surreal, but it was also tangible and yet..... Was it even possible? Am I crazy?" The odor of my brother still lingered in the air, and I could feel his presence near me. I know it was real, but it wasn't possible. "I will give my mother the message and never speak of this again. Everyone will think I'm crazy, if I tell anyone," I thought.

Was God telling me that Daryl is in heaven? Was it real? I have never heard of such a thing happening to anyone.

There was a tapping on my bedroom window, and I heard somebody call, "Judith, wake up!" I glanced at the clock. It was 5:14 a.m.

"Judith, Its Kris, I need to talk to you," she hollered.

I invited Kris and her friend Sam, to come inside. Sam gave her a ride to my house, from Beaumont. "Can we go in your room and speak privately?" Kris asked me.

Kris confided that she had been out all night and was having an affair with her new girlfriend, Sam. I asked her to consider the pain and betrayal she was bringing to her family, not to mention her eternal life. I gently rebuked and corrected her with the word of God, before returning to the living room. We read a bit from the bible and I prayed with them both. I made Kris promise to go directly home before she and Sam drove away.

Within the hour following Kris's departure, I received a phone call from a man.

"Is this Judith?"

"Yes, this is Judith. May I ask who is calling?"

The stranger introduced himself as a neighbor to Kris and Andy. He asked if I knew where Kris was and I told him that she had just left here.

"Judith, do you know where she went? There has been a tragic accident this morning and I need to find Kris as quickly as possible," he informed me.

"She promised me she would go home, about an hour ago," I told him

"Andy is dead," he divulged hesitantly. "He turned his gun on himself, killing himself in front of their two children while they sat watching cartoons on the television," he said. "CPS is here and they will take her children if I don't find her."

"I think I might know where she is. Give me a few minutes to find her."

In our conversation that morning, Kris had told me about the motel she and Sam stayed at the night before. I drove to the motel and found the familiar car that had been parked in my driveway earlier that morning.

I yelled Kris's name and she came running to me.

"What are you doing here, Judith," she asked.

"You need to go home right now! You promised me you would go right home. There is no easy way to tell you this, but Andy has shot and killed himself. CPS is there with the police and will take your children if you don't return home immediately. This is not a game anymore and playtime is over Kris. Do you understand me," I said scorning her.

I returned home and attempted to locate Michael, to tell him of Andy's demise, but he was nowhere to be found.

The days passed, and all I could dwell on was the multitude of recent tragedies in my life. I was lost, alone and confused, feeling the need to take control of my own life. I wept before God until I was completely undone. I was afraid to put a voice to the words that were filling my heart. My tears raged like an uncontrolled river, flowing from my eyes and my hands trembled with fear.

"One tragedy after another has struck me, Lord. Serving You has opened the flood gates to attacks from the enemy and you have failed to protect me," I said relating my life to Job.

I cried out over a period of several days, begging, demanding, manipulating, and arguing my case before Jesus, hoping He would step in and change my life, to make everything right again.

"You're not helping me Lord, and You are not listening to me either. I can't do this anymore. Do You hear me? No more," I sobbed, completely broken and feeling hopeless.

"I'm turning my back on You now, Jesus, just like You've done to me, and I'm walking away quietly. I love you with all my heart, but I can't do this anymore. I've had enough. I won't serve You anymore. If You won't fight for me, then I'll fight for myself and my children, all alone."

I turned my back, and took three steps, to symbolically turn myself away from the dangers of serving God, packed my bags and left California, only to return months later.

Our children were growing fast, and the time flew by very quickly. I remembered an old cliché my mother used to speak to me. "When the going gets tough, the tough get going, and I was going at full speed.

I found a job in a small diner in Torrance, working full time, over time, and all the time I could get. I worked side jobs and made crafts to earn extra money. I worked seven days a week, and 12 to 18 hours a day to make ends meet. I worked hard, lived hard, and loved hard, to give my children a better chance at life.

I walked in prideful determination, keeping God and church out of our lives, always staying one step ahead of God.

I partnered Jimmy, making him the little man of the house, causing him to grow up quickly. He assumed the role of leadership, acting out in his own rebellious anger. He was becoming physically violent toward other young men his age, who did not yield to his control. He used his leadership role to further and strengthen his own self-generated entitlements, for personal rights and gain.

Jeffrey withdrew deeper and deeper into his own little world, escaping reality. While, Jeni-lee became angry and rebelled against everyone, and everything. Her voice and her demands were loud and clear.

Jeni-lee carried her acting out to school. I received a request from her teacher to come to school for two weeks with her, to observe her. I explained that I was a single working parent, living paycheck to paycheck and couldn't do it. Her teacher refused to accept my inability to do so. She said she would fail Jeni-lee if I refused, and she did.

I started getting phone calls twice a week, at work. Each time, Jeni-lee had a temperature of 99 F, and the school demanded that I come pick her up. I had to bring her to work with me, which only encouraged her to continue in her behavior.

I returned from work one afternoon to learn that she had attempted to jump from her second story bedroom window. I immediately enrolled her in counseling.

Jeni-lee complained I was never home, she didn't have any friends at school and everyone made fun of her. She insisted she was stupid, horribly ugly, and nobody cared about her, and even her dad had left her.

I continued Jeni-lee's counseling and involved her in other programs such as ballet, music lessons and art, in an attempt to build her confidence.

I started to search for the perfect man, who would be a good husband and caring father to my children, hoping that a father image would bring her comfort.

My relationships with the new men in my life turned out to be short term relationships, mostly resulting in alcoholics prone to physical violence.

The last boyfriend resulted in battery, stalking and a restraining order to protect my children as well as myself.

I lost my jobs as a result of a work related injury, leaving me with extreme weakness on my right side, and I survived by collecting workers compensation.

I met another beau and we all moved together to a more affordable community, in Yucca Valley where I enrolled my children in school and immediately found a counselor for my daughter.

The alcohol and abuse continued with my newest boyfriend and the phone calls from the school, pertaining to Jeni-lee continued.

I started preparing an early dinner, when the phone rang. It was the school calling to offer their condolences on the loss of my brother, Kurt Cobain, of Nirvanna.

"Who? I've never heard of Kurt Cobain. Who is he?" I asked confused.

She calmly told me that Jeni-lee had been crying in class and said she was sad because your brother, and her uncle, Kurt Cobain had died, but you made her go to school anyway.

The school suggested a meeting and counseling for my daughter. I explained to them that she was already in counseling.

The days passed and the school called to ask for another meeting with me. This time, she had reported that someone had touched her inappropriately.

I returned home with Jeni-lee and began questioning her. I asked her to tell me everything. Her story completely changed four times within an hour. None of them making any sense. This had become far too serious and was no longer one of her entertaining anecdotes. I needed to know the truth. I called Loma Linda Behavioral Clinic to make an appointment for my daughter and threw my boyfriend out.

Jeni-lee spent more than a month in the Loma Linda Clinic before they called me to release her. It was of their professional opinion that she had not been molested and said she had been diagnosed with mild psychosis.

They continued to explain, telling me that when I would say something to Jeni-lee, she would reinterpret my words and that is what she would believe I said or happened. I was advised to be very patient with her.

The doctors had prescribed three medications for her, warning me not give her any other medication, not even Tylenol while she took these. The result could be death, they warned.

I watched her closely and returned her to school. The medications were slowly making her emotionally non-existent. She had morphed into an empty shell, never smiling, or speaking, and just stared off into space.

Soon, it was spring again and the phone rang as a cool breeze blew in through an open window. It was the school, asking me to come immediately. Jeni-lee had been in a fight. Another student had relentlessly teased her, and she hurt the other little girl bad enough to be taken to the doctor to be checked.

"We know Jeni-lee is under counseling and on medication. We want you to consider increasing her medications to keep her calmer," the teacher said.

Her words stuck me like a knife in my heart. "I have complied with everything you have asked of me. I put my daughter in both private and family counseling and even went so far as, to admit her into Loma Linda Behavioral Clinic for more than a month. I even allowed them to put her on some very dangerous, addictive medications that have nearly put her in an emotional comatose state. Any increase will put her down for the count and I won't have it," I sternly told her.

"You are allowing the children in this school to continually bully my daughter in a relentless, unforgiving manner. If my daughter, being nearly a zombie on this medication, snapped and beat the hell out of another girl, then she probably pushed Jeni-lee to do it, and you weren't doing your job and supervising the students," I snapped at them. "Maybe you should be calling the other parents," I yelled as I stood to walk away.

Jeni-lee asked to go to a slumber party at her neighbor and friend's house. I gave my permission, and she left for Brandy's home across the street.

Jeni-lee returned home worn out, the next morning and crawled into her bed.

Brandy's mom came to see me while Jeni-lee slept, to tell me of an incident, the night before.

"The girls were in the kitchen making a snack. I walked in to see Jeni-lee had made a couple of lines from flour, mimicking cocaine, and took a straw from my kitchen drawer and snorted the flour up her nose. I just thought you should know."

"Thank you for telling me," I said walking her to the door.

I questioned Jeni-lee and she confided that she tried to do what she had seen on television and snorted some flour to mimic them. We had a serious talk. Fearful that she may try drugs, and knowing it would threaten her life while taking her prescriptions, I stopped all medications. Before long, her beautiful, vibrant personality returned.

Finally I had met a really nice man who treated me and my children well. He was kind and generous. We dated for several months before Mike had asked me to marry him and to Colorado to become a family. I left my children with my mother and followed him to Colorado to get established and settled before returning for my children. The day had finally come. As he secured the house and property, I returned to California to pack up my children and tie up every loose end.

We telephoned back and forth to each other for three or four days before it happened. I called him and there was no answer. He had disappeared with all my clothes, my truck, my money and had stolen six thousand dollars from my mother's credit card which she expected me to pay back every penny, and rightfully so.

My SSDI claim had been denied. I had lost everything, and wondered how I would ever recover from this mishap.

We stayed with my mother and I fell into a heavy depression. She was very angry, with a deep seeded grievance toward me, and bitterness had crept into her heart.

I borrowed a pretty yellow dress from her and went out that evening with every intention of killing myself. "Maybe now someone will step up to care for my children, because I can't," I murmured in self-pity.

I awoke the following morning, nude, laying in a pool of dried blood, on the floor of an old abandoned house.

Not knowing where I was, I looked around at the piles of trash, attempting to locate my clothing. I reached for my dress, carefully slipping it back on. I slowly lifted myself to my feet, feeling dizzy and unstable. There was garbage everywhere. I saw a bathroom adjacent from me. There was a broken mirror in front of me, surrounded by walls that were smeared with feces, and garbage strewn everywhere. I looked at myself in the broken mirror to see a large hole in my forehead. My face was covered in the brownish red, dried blood. A clear fluid flowed from the new wound in my forehead, mingling with a fresh, bright red blood. My entire face was swollen and puffy with my eyes nearly swollen shut.

"I guess I'm still alive," I dismally thought to myself, embarrassed at my failure to commit suicide. The front of my mother's dress was no longer yellow. The blood had soaked into the fabric, turning it a rust color. I vaguely remembered someone striking me with an object.

I ran water into the dirty, clogged sink that was walled with dirty, menstrual napkins, moldy food, empty beer cans, bugs and various kinds of trash. I unsuccessfully, attempted to wash the blood from my face without touching anything.

I stepped over the garbage, filling the floor and walked into what was once a living room. I found an elderly, homeless man, sitting in a chair that the stuffing had been ripped out of.

"Where am I?" I watched him shrug his shoulders at me, never saying a word.

"Can you tell me where the I-10 is from here?" I asked.

Without a word, he pointed to the broken front door, hanging on one hinge, never looking up from the can of beer he cupped in his hands.

I walked through the front door, feeling the liquid and fresh blood trickling down my face. I looked over the empty fields and saw a freeway not far away. Recognizing the signs, I realized it was the I-10. I walked down a dirt road until I found pavement. My lips were dry and I was very thirsty when I spotted a Circle K, near the freeway onramp.

I walked into the convenience store, uncomfortably aware of every eye turned toward me, with expressions of shock. I set a Pepsi on the counter and asked the cashier where I was. With a look of shock, he stuttered, "Calimesa."

I left the store and continued south to the I-10 onramp, praying a police officer didn't drive by as I put my thumb out for a ride.

"Please God, help me get a ride quickly," I whispered.

The first two vehicles turned sideways to get a better look at me as they drove past. The third vehicle stopped and gave me a ride. He was a kind gentleman, who drove me right to my mother's door, several miles away.

I returned home to my children and the Lord convicted my heart for what I had done. For the first time in my life, I felt the discipline of a true loving Father. I returned to church with my children where we celebrated Jeni-lee's thirteenth birthday with a cake and a party, given by the members at church. One Sunday morning, while in church, the Lord healed my entire right side, and I was hired with my very first job application and returned to work. My mother helped me with transportation to and from work until I saved enough money for a down payment on a used car.

One evening, I received a phone call at work, telling me Jeni-lee had run away from home. I returned home, and called the police to report her as a runaway.

The days turned to weeks and I was finally able to rent an apartment for Jeffrey, and myself. I had met another man, Rodney, and began to date him.

One afternoon while driving Jeffrey to his friend's house, he yelled, "There's Jeni-lee!"

I looked up to see three girls standing in a drive way. "Where, Jeffrey? I don't see her anywhere," I said, searching for her.

"Right there! She is standing right there in front of you, mom," he said, frustrated.

I looked into the face of one of the young ladies standing in front of me, realizing it was Jeni-lee. She stood 5' 6" and weighed, maybe 65 lbs., with a skeletal appearance. Her hair was gone. She was bald with only a few sparse strands of long hair in various areas of the top of her head. Acne had covered her face and I was barely able to recognize my own daughter.

Astonished at the sight of her, I drove around the corner, throwing my hands over my face and began to sob vehemently. Tweaking on methamphetamines and other drugs caused her to pull her hair out, one strand at a time, until she was nearly completely bald.

I returned to the place where I had last seen her and took her home with me to stay. It wasn't long, before she ran away, and disappeared again.

The years were passing and Jeffrey moved out on his own while I worked and continued to live life on my own.

One morning at work, I had received an urgent call. It was Jeffrey, "Mommmm," the world slowly tumbled from his lips as he wept, struggling for his next breath. He fought his emotions, attempting to vocalize his next words. "My Aunt just called and said my dad's dead," he cried out.

I found Jeni-lee and told her that her father had died, and then I phoned Jimmy in Oklahoma to tell him the bad news. The four of us began our mourning of Michael's death that day.

The following March, Jimmy returned for a weeklong visit, bringing with him, my first born grandchild, Brandon. He was incredible and Jimmy's identical twin. I reveled in the beauty and perfection of the newest edition to my family and simultaneously, I mourned, realizing Michael would never see, or know his grandchildren. Jimmy returned to Oklahoma with his new family, only to return to California a year later, after separating from his girlfriend.

Shortly after Jimmy's return home, my mother suffered a massive heart attack, encumbering me with her care. She had appointed me as her "Medical Power of Attorney," and I continued to provide for, and care for her.

Meanwhile, Jeffrey had fallen into a deep depression, following his father's death. He turned to drugs and became suicidal. Fearful for his life, I asked Jimmy to take him in and help me to guide him back to a life of meaningful sobriety in the real world, in today's society.

Before long, my current relationship had crumbled, and I fell into another relationship, still searching for that "someone" to love me. Valentine's Day had arrived, and my new beau had planned a motorcycle adventure through Joshua Tree National Park. We journeyed out on his beautiful, modified Valkyrie 1500, with the saddle bags packed for a romantic picnic.

Suddenly, there were the sounds of sirens screeching through the cool breeze, as I lay in the remnants of my shattered helmet, with shards of the face plate, piercing through my forehead, cheek, teeth and tongue. An ambulance transported my broken, limp body to Desert Regional Trauma Unit. I found myself lying in the very same room that my brother Daryl had been treated in so many years before. I suffered torn ligaments, a broken wrist, brain injury, short and long term memory loss, broken and missing teeth, along with plenty of cuts, requiring stitches about my head and face. My new beau had sprained his ankle in the accident, and we quit dating.

It was a Sunday afternoon, and Mother's Day. I returned home from work to see the red light blinking on my answering machine. The message was from Jeni-lee. She was screaming hysterically, begging me to return her call.

She answered the phone and cried for me to listen to her and wanted to know if she could come home. "I promise to stop drugs, mom. It just hit me, my dad is dead and if you die too, I won't have anyone left to care about me. Please, mom!"

It was the greatest Mother's Day gift I would ever receive! I brought her home, took her job hunting, and enrolled her in C.N.A. classes. She was working part time and attending school, when she started to drink. I told her that her behavior would stop immediately, or she would have to move out, hoping to threaten her back to her senses.

One afternoon, I received a call at work from Jeni-lee. She had something very urgent to discuss with me. She sounded frightened and distressed and asked me to hurry home.

I rushed home, only to find her gone. She was nowhere to be found, but all her clothing was still there. I diligently searched for her for a week. She had vanished into thin air without a word or a trace. Frightened for her, I filed a missing person's report.

Nearly a month passed before receiving a phone call from the Banning Police Department. The officer told me they had found a body, matching the general description of my daughter, Jeni-lee, and asked for identifying marks or tattoos.

"She talked about getting a tattoo, but I don't know if she did, or not," I replied

The investigating officer said she would call back once they made a determination, or knew more.

I called her brothers to question them about tattoos, and they didn't know any more than I did. Before I knew it, Jimmy and Jeffrey barreled through my front door.

"Did you hear anything yet?" Jeffrey asked.

"Not yet. I'm still waiting," I said nervously pacing.

Nearly four hours passed as we sat on the edge of our seats, ready to lunge at the first ring of the phone, or knock on the door. Fear and dread overwhelmed us as we sat, impatiently waiting.

"I'm not waiting any longer. I'm going to call, and if they don't tell me anything, I am going down there to see for myself," I railed with fierce determination as I dialed the number.

"This is Ms. Birdsong. I haven't heard from you in several hours. Do I need to come down to identify the body?" I said gripping the receiver tightly, in an effort to salvage any sanity that I had left.

"We have identified the body and it's not your daughter. We will keep searching for her and notify you when we find her," The officer reported.

Jimmy and Jeffrey fell back against the sofa in relief. We spent some time together, comforting each other before they began their journey back home.

Weeks later, a Los Angeles Police officer identified himself on the phone and said, he had found Jeni-lee asleep on the beach.

"Your daughter is very ill and refuses medical attention," he told me, before putting her on the phone.

I begged her to go to the hospital, and offered to pick her up. She abruptly said she was fine and would call me later, before she hung up on me.

Months had passed since that dreadful call from LAPD, before Jeni-lee called me. She had hitchhiked to Missouri to see family. While staying with her cousin, Lindsey, she had fallen and struck her head. Refusing medical attention, she complained of severe swelling and headaches, pleading for a bus ticket to come home.

I agreed, purchased a bus ticket for her, and made arrangements to pick her up at the terminal.

Jeni-lee's drinking spiraled out of control. It occurred to me, to do the same thing I had done with Jeffrey. I sent her away, to stay with Jimmy to separate her from her poor choice of friends and connections.

A year later, I walked the hospital corridors with Jeni-lee to regulate her labor pains.

I stood next to the doctor watching, as my incredible granddaughter fought her way into the world. Aryana Lee was as beautiful as her mother, the day I gave birth to her.

"If only Michael were here to see this stunning and amazing little creature, who looked exactly like him. Immediately, I saw that her physical appearance was a female Michael. I held her against my heart in the delivery room as my heart melted inside of me.

Aryana was a week old when Jeni-lee called me, asking me to come and get her. She was breaking up with her boyfriend. I moved my two girls in with me that very day, and Jeni-lee quickly found a new beau.

Aryana was three months old, when Jeni-lee announced that she was pregnant. She asked me if she should get an abortion. Not knowing what to say to her, I told her that it wasn't my decision to make, but I didn't agree that abortion was an answer. After the doctor confirmed her pregnancy, the boyfriend left, abandoning her and their unborn child.

Before long, I was standing beside the doctor once more, watching another beautiful granddaughter fight her way into this world. Savannah Lee looked more like me than she did her grandfather, with a hint of her father in her. Now, I had the joy of all three of my girls living with me, and my life was good!

Jeni-lee met an old friend, and moved in with him, taking my precious granddaughters with her.

Before long, I started dating Brian, who lived about 45 minutes from me. I would often stay the weekend with him, because of the distance. Lately, I had been feeling very weak, dizzy, and short of breath, most of the time. I fought to hide it from others, feeling the pull of God on my life once more.

I prayerfully explained to Jesus, I was still too afraid to follow Him, in light of the horrific events of my past, and I still didn't believe, or trust that He would protect me.

I left for Lawndale, to spend a weekend with my closest friend and confidant, Debbie. We sat outside one evening while I confided that I knew, I was going to die, and it would be soon. It was just a feeling I had, but I knew. I asked her to pray in agreement with me, that God would not let me go to hell. Afterwards, I returned home to see my granddaughters, Aryana, who had recently turned three years old, and Savannah who was two.

I waited in Brian's home, while he drove to San Diego to finish up a job. I telephoned Debbie to tell her I was having difficulty breathing, and I was afraid I was going to die. Brian received mail at a P.O. Box and I couldn't find anything with a physical address on it to call 911. There was no landline and I became increasingly alarmed as

Debbie encouraged me to stay calm. I hung up and called Brian to tell him I needed to go to the ER. He started home immediately, while unsuccessfully trying to reach 911 from his cell phone.

An hour later, Brian drove me a block and a half to the local fire station. I was transported by ambulance, to the nearest hospital.

After spending three days on life support, I opened my eyes and searched my environment. I found my mother, my children, some of my siblings, Debbie and her daughter, Autumn, surrounding my bed.

My first conscious thought was, "Oh my God, I could be burning in hell right now," realizing my second chance! At that very moment, I gave my life back to Jesus Christ.

I learned that I had suffered respiratory exacerbation, bringing about complete respiratory failure. Apparently, when I had quit smoking cold turkey, my body went into shock from the withdrawals and shut down. Slowly I was removed from the C-PAP as they continued to heavily medicate me over the next two weeks, before releasing me.

The pain in my body increased as did the severe weakness, and I remained undiagnosed, despite every test that was performed. For the first time in my life, I was speedily gaining weight and none of my clothes fit me any longer. I continued to push forward, believing God would heal me.

I was no longer able to work and without a diagnosis, I was unable to collect any form of disability. In no time at all, I lost my home, car, bank account, credit, as well as, almost everything else I owned, including all my clothes and shoes. The pain had become unbearable and I was dependent on Brian for a place to live.

While I stayed with Brian, Jeni-lee called me to ask if I would take Aryana and Savannah to live with me, while she sorted out her relationship problems with her boyfriend. The girls stayed with me for a time, before their mother returned to pick them up.

I was barely able to stand or walk and no longer able to stoop over and lift my body back up on my own. The pain and weakness in my body had become excruciatingly debilitating.

Brian and I were no longer getting along and it was time for me to move along. I met a woman in Yucca Valley who invited me to stay with her and her husband. In that year, the Lord God healed me enough to stand and move around for short periods of time. After spending more than three years in bed undiagnosed, and on a very slow road to recovery, I was incredibly excited and thankful.

I spent the next year living in a small store room in the back of a thrift store and volunteered in a Domestic Violence Shelter, until I was hired as a child/teen advocate. The Lord used my time there to teach me and open my eyes through revelation pertaining to my life.

The Domestic Violence Shelter had no more than dissolved my position as child/teen advocate, laying me off, when out of the blue, , Jeni-lee called me. I had only seen Aryana and Savannah a couple of times in the past two years and had few phone conversations with them. Jeni-lee said that she wanted to seek professional help for her drinking, and asked me to take the girls while she worked out her problems.

During their stay, Aryana had confessed to me about a man who had tried to touch her, in a way he shouldn't. She said that she got away from him and he didn't hurt her. I immediately called Jeni-lee and told her what Aryana had told me, along with the man's first name. I told her to call the police and report him, since I didn't know who, or where this man was. She cried and agreed to take care of it right away.

I returned to my granddaughters to assure them that they were very good girls and had done nothing wrong. I promised them that mommy and I would make sure nothing like this would ever happen to them again.

Weeks later, Jeni-lee returned to take her daughters home with her.

I had been living in the Thrift store for a year and managed to save enough money to buy a used vehicle with the help of my son, Jeffrey. For the first time in years, I was mobile again.

The thrift store had been sold and it was time for me to move on, once again. I was approved for unemployment and stayed with my son, Jeffrey and his wife, while I searched for employment and another place to live.

Chapter 9
An Emotional Healing

Without interruption He continued,

"Judith, my daughter, I have heard your cries, and I have loved you so very much. I have spent these years calling for you to return to Me."

He spoke again saying,

"You chose to spend these years in rebellion against Me. Do you remember so many years ago, when you became angry with Me? When you unrighteously judged Me, ….. Me, God? You turned your back on me and walked away, blaming Me for your various trials and losses, brought upon you, by your own lack of knowledge, your rebellion, and your sins! When you did this, My daughter, you took your children with you. You removed them out from under the umbrella of My protection, along with yourself,"

He whispered to me with such a depth of love.

"Because you have asked Me, I am faithful to forgive. Because you have invited Me, I am faithful to return. Because you have inquired of Me, I am faithful to answer, and because you have petitioned Me, I am faithful to save."

Jesus continued to confirm to me…..

"Follow Me, and I will show you how you have opened the doors for evil to overtake you and your children, that you may understand. Follow me now that I may teach you how to close these doors. You will learn and understand my precepts. Come with Me now, my daughter, to the beginning. Let Me show you what you did wrong. Do you remember these great many years ago, when you kneeled beside your bed in prayer, and you held a knife to your heart…..

I closed my eyes and the memories of the events in a life gone by, began to flood and fill every chamber of my heart and mind. In the twinkle of an eye, Jesus had taken me back through the years of my past and shown me, my great and many trials and sins over the past 40 years. Unexpectedly, there it was….. "The Truth!" It lay bare before me and yet I knew there was still so much more than what I was seeing. Bitter memories of my abortion and the attempted abortion of my daughter, Jeni-lee began to flood my mind. My eyes were wide open and suddenly, I understood. My memories consumed me as I realized that I had emotionally aborted, my children, my family, and my friends, but I had especially aborted my daughter emotionally, while she lay in my womb.

I had built a very high wall of protection and held it up with a stronghold that nobody was able to penetrate. A shameful sadness and grief fell upon my broken heart and my pride crumbled, leaving a small hole, or gap in the wall of protection, I had struggled so hard to erect.

I continued to ponder upon the memories of so very long ago, in the dark and dreary times of my life. My thoughts overflowed with memories of grief, fear, rejection and confusion. It seemed as though it were another person in another lifetime. I knew it was time to act and I had to do something, but what? Somehow this wretched life of mine had become my testimony and I knew that I had to help educate others so they would not make the same mistakes that I had made.

Suddenly, I heard that still, quiet voice again. The small voice echoed, *"Write it all down!"*

I opened my eyes and the memories of my obstinacy and rebellion unfolded as a greater understanding, and revelation of His promise to deliver, teach and heal me flooded my very soul. Truth overwhelmed me and the reality of my own life struck me so hard that it awoke me to a knowledge of His great wisdom. It was then that I recalled the prophetic words in Isaiah 48 that were given to me when I was pregnant with Jeni-lee.

As I wrote on a notebook that lay near me, the tears of conviction, remorse, and grief flowed as I felt the bricks, one by one, start to tumble and fall. The anguish that arose through repentance for my past misdeeds and the bitter regrets flooded my heart. The awareness of the pain, and grief I had brought upon others that I loved so dearly, had overcome my senses. The wall that I had so perfectly and painstakingly erected for the protection of my heart and my livelihood was tumbling down…. Brick by brick by brick… With every brick that came tumbling down, Jesus was able to move in that much closer to me and finally, He became my protection and a new trust formed and grew for Him.

I wrote everything down, finally realizing that it was all leading back to the abortion, I'd had 40 years earlier.

The battle for my daughter and my granddaughters had only just begun. Jeni-lee drowned herself in drugs and alcohol to numb her pain in a way that I had never seen before. Eventually she disappeared and I continued my visits with Aryana and Savannah.

I decorated the extra bedroom of my two bedroom home, enrolled in parenting classes, and applied for, and was approved for foster parenting, in Hopes of gaining custody of my granddaughters. I attended every court hearing. I had no finances for an attorney and hoped the judge would hear me. I complied with everything that CPS asked and required of me. I wrote letters to several attorneys, pleading for help, pro bono, and to no avail. I continued to pray and fast, standing in faith for God's supernatural miracles. I knew in my heart of hearts, that I was doing everything possible to gain full custody of the two little girls that I loved more than my own life. After all, I am their mother too, just once removed.

The months passed and we lost the battle to regain custody. Aryana and Savannah were adopted, leaving me with no further contact or visitations.

I was devastated and distraught at the final loss. I couldn't take anymore loss. I felt as though I had been broken beyond the point of ever healing again, and I struggled to hold on to my faith.

I sat at my kitchen table, downcast and praying, when the phone rang. I answered to hear a child's faint whisper, "Grandma!"

"Aryana!" I called out in surprise. "Where are you?"

"Grandma, I'm at school, and I wanted to call you to tell you that I love you grandma," she whispered faintly. "I told the nurse, I didn't feel good and I wanted to call my mom. I sneaked to call you, grandma. I can't talk very loud or they will hear me," she secretly voiced.

"I'm so happy you called me. I miss you so much Aryana. Do you know how much I love you and your sister too? I love you so much! You are my precious angel, Aryana, never forget that," I voiced in a miserable, failed attempt to hide the breaks in my voice as the tears flowed from my eyes.

"I love you too, grandma! Are you crying? Why are you crying, grandma?"

"Oh, these are my happy tears, baby girl! I am just so happy that you called me," I replied. "Is your adopted mom going to let me see you? Can we visit each other, Aryana? Tell her you want to visit me," I struggled with my broken words and fragmented heart.

"No, grandma. They won't let me see you again," she answered as her voice stretched out into long inflections of a weary sadness. Grandma, I have to go now, but I just wanted to say good bye and tell you that I really, really love you, grandma! Please don't cry grandma. I love you grandma, good by….. And grandma….. God bless you, grandma," she said, her words crumbled, permanently finalizing our conversation. She hung up the phone, and my wounded spirit cried out.

I gripped the phone tightly between my fingers as I folded my arms across the table and laid my head down on my arms where I wept profusely for an undetermined amount of time.

I continued on to church one Sunday, and heard the Pastor announce that Laura Jensen was here today from the High Desert Pregnancy Clinic. He announced that anyone wanting to speak with her, should see her in the back after services.

I spoke with Laura immediately after services and she referred me to the clinic.

On Monday, the very next afternoon, I went to the clinic where I met a P.A.R. (Post Abortive Recovery) counselor, Glenda Machado. I explained to her that I was writing a book and needed more information about abortion.

The lovely and sweet young woman questioned me, "Have you ever had an abortion Judith?" Her voice was very soft, laced with a tender compassion.

"Yes, when I was sixteen I had one. It was a very long time ago," I said in an attempt to turn the conversation back to the present to gather needed information from her. I am feeling led of God, to write a book, exposing the full scope of the atrocities that abortion brings into the lives of post abortive women, using my own life as a testimony and example," I said trying to smile.

"Judith, have you ever received, 'Post Abortive Counseling'? Perhaps you would consider going through our grief counseling course with me? You would learn a lot about what we do here and perhaps it would even help you to have a greater understanding of what has happened to you. It may even help you to write your book," Glenda smiled with such a tender kindness.

"No, I've never had post abortive counseling," I answered anxiously. "Well, my abortion was so long ago, I'm sure I've already dealt with it. I'm okay, but you're right, it would probably help me to learn a lot more about the subject," I replied. Together we set a schedule that would be convenient for both of us, and planned my first appointment.

The course with Glenda had begun and so had the healing process. I examined every brick I had used to build my wall of protection. I found that each brick, was wholly comprised of labeled emotions, such as guilt, grief, fear, pain, and anger. For the first time in my life, I saw the tremendous amount of unrecognized and undiagnosed grief that I had been suffering from, for so many years.

I reflected upon a question my mother had asked me many years ago. She asked, "Judith, what has happened to you, to make you so hard?"

Finally, I had an answer to that question. I only wish my mother were still alive, so I could share my answer with her. The answer is "For forty years, I have been walking in a fog, blind and without understanding. I was filled with: Guilt, Grief, Shame, Pain, Anger, Fear, Confusion, Disillusionment, and last, but not least, Uncertainty.

It is time for the fog to lift, allowing the 'SON'shine to break through and the long process of healing to begin. A couple of years have passed since counseling with Glenda and the healing process is not completely finished, yet. I don't know that it ever will be, but I get a little bit better every day. It seems to come in layers, a little at a time, as understanding fills my body, spirit and soul. It is time for me to stop being the 'Post Abortive Woman,' and become the 'Emotionally Healed Woman', who had an abortion.

After writing these pages, I am just beginning to understand the depth of the emotional abortion I have set over my subsequent children, especially my daughter. I have come to understand that an emotional abortion extended far beyond, just the reaches of my children, but also, to my husband, my marriage, and virtually every other relationship throughout my life.

I have come to believe that even those who do not abort an unwanted pregnancy, choosing to keep the baby, have already emotionally aborted it, even though they have loved it from the moment it was born. I believe the unborn child inherits a spirit of rejection, death and even murder, in the womb and continues to act out in rebellion and anger after birth. Often times it results in teen age pregnancy, adolescent drug use, or addiction, or gang related adolescent activity, leading to young adults, who continue to drink the bitter waters of life, for reasons that we have not understood.

I believe that because I walked in the grief filled fog, that was ignited by my abortion, and because of my efforts to abort my pregnancy when I carried Jeni-lee, I caused her to not only inherit the spirit of rejection, but also the spirit of murder that led her to self-mutilation and multiple attempts to commit suicide. Because she is an adult, making her own choices, all that is left for me to do now is to pray, and believe God for her healing and deliverance as I continue to love her unconditionally.

Through the professional counseling of Glenda Machado and the wonderful support I received at the High Desert Pregnancy Clinic, I discovered that I have been suffering from P.A.S. (Post Abortive Syndrome) and its various symptoms for 40 years. Some of these symptoms for me, were (but not limited to);

1. Grief
2. Low Self Esteem
3. Depression/Anger, though often buried deeply
4. Guilt
5. Alienation from self, family, friends & others
6. Isolation
7. Nightmares/Baby Dreams
8. Sleep Disorders
9. Suicidal Thoughts
10. Relationship Problems; 70% of romantic relationships end after an abortion. Some women also distance themselves from their nuclear family and from their closest friends.
11. Intimacy Problems; Women often shy away from intimate relationships with males for fear of having to reveal things about herself, including her abortion.
12. Physical Pain; Women may describe pain such as abdominal pain, menstrual pain, or back pain. This

could be organic pain caused by complications from the abortion or it could be psychosomatic pain.

13. Hyper Alertness
14. Difficulties in subsequent pregnancies, labor and delivery, such as labor that starts and stops or that fails to progress resulting in cesareans.
15. Inability to bond properly with subsequent children. The bond that does develop is characterized by overly protective behavior and emotional distancing.
16. Avoidance Behavior centered on children, pregnancy and abortion.
17. Eating disorders
18. Sexual dysfunction or promiscuity
19. Atonement Pregnancy: feeling compelled to become pregnant again, often within one year following the abortion
20. Abusive Relationships: In some cases, the woman is the abusive party, in other cases she is the abused party
21. Spiritual Wounds: for many women this may be the first experience of "serious sin." Some women fear that God will punish them, especially when it comes to future childbearing experiences.
22. Increased bitterness toward men: this manifests itself in terms of being able to really trust men in the future.
23. Involvement with pro-life movement or pro-abortion movements.

(For a more detailed list of symptoms: See my Workbook, "An Emotional Healing," coming soon.)

There are indeed, more symptoms than what is curtailed in this list, however, these are the predominate symptoms that addressed me. While every symptom listed above has affected me, the two symptoms that seemed to stand out, above all others, are numbers 1. Grief, and 15. The inability to bond properly with my subsequent children, but I will come back to these two later. First I would like to identify and share with you, how the other symptoms have affected my life after abortion.

1. Grief: For explanation, see below
2. Low Self-esteem: I felt a hollow emptiness within the very center of my existence. I no longer felt worthy of love, compassion, or forgiveness. I believed that I had let everyone down and I had failed both, Jesus and my mother, the two most important people in my life.
3. Depression/Anger, though often buried deeply: I suffered severe bouts of depression. I stopped talking to others and buried myself in the darkness of my room, by covering my windows with foil. There I could dwell among the tombs of the buried memories that continually haunted me, in the lost and silent ugliness of my life, where anger and rage filled my heart. Words and Sarcasm became my newest choice of weaponry, and with cutting sarcasm, I made the world feel the pangs of my anger and rage. I became a verbal, flesh eating monster.
4. Guilt: I felt guilty for murdering the life of an innocent baby, and not just any baby, but my own baby. A good mother would instinctively protect her child. I felt terribly guilty and abnormal for failing to protect my own, unborn child. I also felt guilty for compromising my own moral beliefs and letting everyone down. My mother had always told me that being the oldest child, I was to be the example to my younger siblings, and I felt guilty for having failed them miserably.
5. Alienation from self, family, friends and others: I would alienate myself emotionally by staying busy all the time so that I wouldn't have to feel pain or sadness anymore. Nobody could penetrate that impenetrable wall that I had erected for myself. Now, nobody could ever hurt me again, not even

me. I had no true friends because I would never let anyone get close enough to me. I was not worthy of their love, their trust, or friendship. I could not trust myself to make educated, intelligent decisions in my life and so, I continued to recklessly, and blindly stab at the winds of a future for myself.

6. Isolation: I isolated myself and my every emotion. I was told by so many that I had a great poker face, therefore, nobody would every truly know or hurt me again. Thus, they would have no weaponry in their quiver of armory to assault me with. I would stand as an island, all alone, and hastily greet every challenge that dared to confront me.

7. Nightmares, Baby Dreams: I had repeated dreams of being pregnant. After my atonement pregnancy, I became very fearful of becoming pregnant again. I believed I has to be a perfect mother to make up for murdering my first child. I seriously doubted that I could do this for one child, on along two or more children. I seldom had physical relations with my husband because of the fear of becoming pregnant. This created even further complications in my marriage.

8. Sleep Disorders: I went from a teenager sleeping ten hours a night, and until noon every day, to a woman who restlessly slept at all. I slept in periodicals of two to five hours a night and five hours of sleep would be really sleeping in late. My dreams became vivid memories that I confused with reality at times. I would have to actually stop, focus, and try to remember if it really happened or if it was another crazy dream.

9. Suicidal Thoughts: Not a day passed when I didn't think about killing myself. I didn't think I had the right live or to be happy. I didn't believe I had any value or worth anymore. I certainly didn't believe I had anything to contribute to the all-encompassing good of humanity, or rather, the goodness of life.

After all, I had already murdered, so why not kill myself too? In fact, I made two unsuccessful attempts at suicide, but I won't go into details here.

10. Relationship Problems: I was unable to hold on to a close relationship with anyone. I emotionally separated myself from my siblings as well as every other family member, other than my mother. I still sought approval and acceptance from my mother. I became the one that tested everyone, or anyone who tried to befriend me. I would set up every new relationship to fail as quickly as possible. After all, nobody could attain the standards of perfect loyalty, perfect trust, and perfect truth that I had, through my own wounded-ness come to expect and demand of them.

11. Intimacy Problems: I was unable to achieve a point of intimacy. If I were intimate with anyone, then all my skeletons would come tumbling out of the closet, all at once. Then they would know. They would know the truth about me. They would know, I have faults beyond measure, they would know, I don't deserve to live, they would know, I am unlovable and I don't belong.

12. Physical Pain: I rarely felt physical pain. My emotional pain had by far succeeded any physical pain that would beset me. That being said, however, there was one pain that would take me down every time. That was menstrual pain. After many visits to several doctors, over many years, the cause of this severe cramping was never determined.

13. Hyper Alertness or Hypervigilance: I became a watchman, a guard if you will, against any intruders who may attempt to bring harm to me or mine. I searched vigilantly, criticizing and judging others, while searching for any threats that invaded my environment. I looked for recognizable or familiar sights, sounds, people, behaviors, smells, or anything else that would be reminiscent of a threat.

I sought out the faults of others and was sure to drive them back, or away by hurting them before they could ever hurt me.

14. Difficulties in Subsequent Pregnancies, labor and delivery: I had several miscarriages and three children. Jimmy lay in my birth canal and despite every effort made to push him out, he refused to deliver. They used forceps to deliver and afterward, I had been placed into recovery where I nearly hemorrhaged to death. A nurse found me in recovery, laying in a pool of my own blood, calling STAT. I hovered under the ceiling, watching until I returned to my body. Jeffrey dropped in my fifth month of pregnancy. I managed to carry him to term, only to discover in child birth, he had a twin in a separate water bag that died premature to full development, about the time I dropped, at the five and a half mark. Jeni-lee, well you know her story after reading this book

15. Inability to Bond Properly with subsequent children. The bond that does develop is characterized by overly protective behavior and emotional distancing: For explanation, see below.

16. Avoidance Behavior centered on children, pregnancy and abortion: I avoided my own subsequent children by working as much as possible and staying so busy that I didn't have time for them. I avoided other women's children at all cost. I didn't like being around other women's children and I couldn't stand the sound of a baby's cry. It became like nails on a chalkboard for me and the sound of a crying baby would send me straight into a near convulsive rage. I gave no recognition, thought, or attention to any woman who became pregnant. I came to believe abortion was a woman's right to choose, justifying myself, and gave it no further thought or attention.

17. Eating Disorders: I stopped eating. I only ate when it became necessary to stop myself from passing out. I convinced myself that eating made me lethargic and caused me to lack the strength to continue in the requirements of the day and therefore, I avoided food except when it became a requirement for survival.

18. Sexual Dysfunction or Promiscuity: I began to look for love, approval and deliverance through anyone who would offer it to me, even if it was only for a night. I met Michael and we married. Sexual promiscuity began after our last separation. Once again, I began to search for love in all the wrong ways and all the wrong places.

19. Atonement Pregnancy: I met a young lady who was with child and decided I would feel better about myself if I were to become pregnant again. I set out to get pregnant again and a year and a half later, my very precious, Jimmy was born.

20. Abusive Relationships: I had become so controlling, fearful and angry that over the years, it drew men to me who were looking to tame what appeared to be a wild, and out of control spirit. Me! In my anger and rebellion, the men in my life found it necessary to beat me into submission and as a result, I learned to fight back. Before long, we had both become the abusers, him through his verbal and physical violence and myself through manipulation, control, and verbal violence, or "Sarcasm."

21. Spiritual Wounds: I was spiritually wounded, and believed I had broken all Ten Commandments, set forth by God Himself, and was speedily on the path to Hell. Not only had I broken every commandment, but I had committed the worst of them all, I had murdered my own child. I didn't believe there could be no true forgiveness, for such a one as I had become. I didn't deserve to live, and there wouldn't be any salvation, for me.

22. Increased Bitterness Toward Men: I no longer trusted men to be there for me. I believed all men wanted was sex and would leave all the consequences for me to deal with alone, and I would. I held no man accountable in any relationship since I didn't believe anyone could sincerely love me anyway. I believed all men were just using me for as long as I would let them, and I would use them back for a moment of solace.

23. Involvement with Pro-Life Movement or Pro-Abortion Movement: I am writing this book, and volunteering at a Pro-Life, Christian founded, pregnancy Clinic.

If you take all of the above listed symptoms and combine them, you will find quite a mess, and I had become that mess, literally. I spent most of the past forty years on the run and never allowing the truth to tag me. I had repressed the memory, details, and emotions of my abortion and stuffed them so deep within myself, that it was impossible for truthful information to reach my conscious mind for recognition or understanding. I logically rationalized my abortion by blaming my mother for forcing me to make the decision to abort my baby. The truth is, it was my decision and nobody forced me. I thought I had accepted my abortion, and I believed I was just fine with the decision I made to have that abortion. Eventually I became psychologically numb.

It felt as if a switch had been turned off inside of me, and I could no longer get excited about anything. I was afraid to show any emotion, other than anger. Anger was my new, best friend, from which I drew all my strength.

Needless to say, this created a problem for me. I no longer had the ability to love and engage in a healthy relationship with anyone.

Was I able to love? Was I able to love my children? Absolutely! The question here is, "Was I able to possess a healthy love and relationship for not only myself, but for my children and others as well?" I loved the only way I knew how, from my wounds. I loved my children through those wounds, and in so doing, I wounded them, causing a lot of damage control to focus on today.

There are still two more symptoms, as I have mentioned above that have brought forth a great deal of devastation in my life, and not only mine, but the lives of my children and my surrounding family and friends as well. I will explain the first symptom, which is "GRIEF." It seemed as if, GRIEF was one of the two culprits that went unrecognized, and took hold of my life. I continued to waltz through life, completely unaware of why I was so miserably unhappy. I came to the conclusion and understanding, there was something, terribly wrong with me, but I didn't understand the "What or Why" of it all. I saw counselors over the years and was told that everything I was feeling was a result of an unhappy and insecure childhood and marriage. Perhaps there was some truth in that explanation, but I believe my grief, discontentment and torment began with my abortion.

1. Grief: After I aborted my child, unbeknownst to me, I filled up with grief. With the exception of the phone call I made to my cousin, which consisted of five minutes or less, I did as my mother had instructed me. I never spoke of my abortion or told anyone about it again, until many years had passed. I shoved my GRIEF so far down, that it lay imprisoned in the darkest recesses of the pit of my bowels. I kept myself so busy, moving and running that I never had time to stop and think, on along feel anything. I had children, got married and filled my life with so much drama that there was no time to stop and listen to the cries, or the fearful bemoaning's that struggled to escape the prison I had encased it in, so many years ago.

Grief is a funny thing. In order for me to heal, I needed to first recognize what was happening to me. I also needed the support, comfort, and encouragement of others. I needed enough time to work through my grief since there is no hard and fast timeline, or rule for the healing of grief.

As soon as I thought I had finally worked through it, it would find me again. I have since learned that GRIEF is the proverbial onion, containing innumerable layers. It seems I can only recognize and heal one layer at a time without becoming so overwhelmed that I can no longer function. I do believe however, that I am finally reaching the center core of this onion, called GRIEF.

I would like to reiterate, GRIEF cannot be rushed. It is a process, which takes time and patience, and a well-grounded support system which I have been blessed enough to find through our local High Desert Pregnancy Clinic. Now let's take a closer look at the word, "GRIEF." According to the Free Dictionary, found online, GRIEF is defined as:

1. Deep mental anguish, as that arising from bereavement, or an instance of this
2. Informal Criticism or rude talk.
3. See Synonym, "Regret."

Now let's take a look at the word, "Regret" using the same dictionary, Regret is defined as:

1. A feeling of sorrow, disappointment, distress, or remorse about something that one wishes could be different.
2. A sense of loss and longing for someone or something gone, or passed out of existence
3. To feel sorry, repentant, or upset about
4. To bemoan or grieve the death or loss of
5. A sense of repentance, guilt, or sorrow, as over some wrong done or an unfulfilled ambition
6. A sense of loss or grief

If you look further into the word "GRIEF," you will find it here in Isaiah 53: 4-6. It reads as follows;

"Surely He has borne our griefs and carried our sorrows; yet we esteemed Him stricken, Smitten by God, and afflicted. But He was wounded for our transgressions, He was bruised for our iniquities; the chastisement for our peace was upon Him, and by His stripes we are healed. All we like sheep have gone astray; we have turned, every

one, to his own way; and the Lord has laid on Him the iniquity of us all."

The word "GRIEFS," taken from the Hebrew word, Choliy, (Kholee), is defined as malady, anxiety, calamity, disease, grief, and (is) sick (-ness). Choliy was derived from the root word Chalah (khaw-law'), meaning to be rubbed or worn; hence, to be weak, sick, afflicted, or to grieve, make sick, also to stroke (in flattering), entreat: - beseech, (be) diseased, (put to) grief, be grieved, (be) grievous, infirmity, entreat, lay to, put to pain, be (fall, make) sick, sore, be sorry, a woman in travail, be (become) weak, be wounded.

Strong's Exhaustive Concordance)

In order to more adequately describe and understand exactly what this means, I have defined a description of each word below:

Malady: disease, disorder, ailment, an unwholesome condition.

Anxiety: state of uneasiness, apprehension, as about future events.

Calamity: an even that brings terrible loss, lasting distress, severe affliction, disaster.

Disease: a pathological condition of a part, organ, or system of an organism, resulting from various causes such as infection, genetic defect, or environmental stress, and characterized by an identifiable group of signs and symptoms.

Grief: deep mental anguish as a threat arising from bereavement, a source of deep mental anguish, annoyance or frustration, trouble or difficulty.

Sickness: the condition of being sick, illness, a disease, a malady, nausea, defective or unsound condition.

Sore: painful to touch, tender, causing misery, sorrow, or distress, causing embarrassment or irritation, full of distress, sorrowful, angry, offended.

Sorry: feeling or expressing sympathy, pity or regret, worthless, or inferior, paltry, causing sorrow, grief, or misfortune.

Paltry: lacking in importance or worth, wretched or contemptible.

You can see by the definitions of the word "GRIEFS," as listed above, that just the word "GRIEFS," all alone and of itself has encompassed all (everything) that we have suffered because we chose to abort (extinguish the life of) our child(ren). In Isaiah 53: 4, the word of God has specifically stated that Jesus has already *"borne our griefs"* and carried all our sorrow. It is vital that we take all our grief's, sorrow, and torment, and lay it down at the foot of the cross, giving it all to Jesus. To hold onto these devastating, life altering, and destructive emotions is to say that what Jesus suffered on the cross for you and I, was not enough.

Remember, not only does grief have no timeline, and peels one layer at a time, pain also has many layers as well, and will peel like the proverbial onion, one layer at a time. Your healing may do the same, or it may come all at once, that is between you and God. The end result is, if you are reading this book, your healing has already begun.

Last, but certainly not least, nor a final symptom, but the next symptom, I have listed below. The second unrecognized culprit for me in this journey is number fifteen on the list. The inability to bond properly with subsequent children. I could not find a definition in the dictionary for number fifteen. Instead, I prayed and sought the Lord for an answer

15. The inability to bond properly with subsequent children. The bond that does develop is characterized by overly protective behavior and emotional distancing: I was unable to bond with my children as a normal mother would. I was unable to hold my babies in my arms for feedings, for rocking, for comforting, or for pleasure. I would lay them down and prop their bottles with a pillow for feeding. When they needed comforted, I would lay them next to me and

pat their little back. I was unable to give hugs that lasted more than a mere three or four seconds. I was unable to physically bond with my babies which led to even greater problems with emotional bonding.

Once I came to recognize that I had been unable to physically, and emotionally connect with my children as other mothers did, I understood that I had actually "Emotionally Aborted," my own children. The emotional attachment to my children had been severely weakened by the lack of physical bonding between us. I comprehended, at last, the rejection, abandonment and unworthiness that my own children were suffering, through the affliction of being emotionally aborted by their own mother. While I never had a problem telling my children just how much I loved them, I failed to show my love for them by making them feel safe and protected through the simple means of touching, caressing, or holding them close to me. I failed to embrace my children, body, spirit and soul.

The words I spoke over my children were harsh, demanding, and spoken with an unkind tone. Over the years, I had become a perfectionist, who demanded such a high standard of performance from others, that it was impossible to meet those standards. I eventually came to embrace sarcasm and anger as: "It is just who I am," never realizing the damage I may be inflicting upon the ones I loved the most.

At the time, I desperately tried to convince myself, as well as others, this is just the way God made me. "So, Get Over It!" I didn't believe I could change, or even needed to.

As I continued to pray and seek the Lord for answers, He started the process of slowly changing me, from the inside out, layer by layer. I had asked Him to show me where I failed as a mother, and He was faithful to answer, revealing the hidden things in me. I continued to work through my pain and grief while He gave to me a greater understanding of the simple things like our words, and the power that is behind them. Our words hold the power to destroy, or create as God did when He said in Genesis 1: 3,

Then God said, "Let there be light," and there was light.

The Spirit of the Lord led me to research, the "Butterfly Effect." I investigated this phenomenon and cried out to Him to explain it to me, so that I might understand.

I was reminded by God, of a prophetic word given to me in 1982, by Mary Nell, in our small Cabazon Foursquare Church. Over these great and many years, I have often searched for the meaning of this prophetic word for me. Once more, I heard the small quiet voice as it said aloud, "Search the words, using the Strong's Exhaustive Concordance." I did so, word by word, and underlined the definition of the words in Isaiah 48: 3-11, 17-18. Finally, it all made perfect sense to me, and I understood the "What and Why's" of it all…..

3. "I have declared the former things from the beginning; They went forth from my *****mouth** (by means of blowing, a small wind, a spoken word, a command and an appointment) and I caused them to **hear it** (to hear intelligently, to give attention to, to be obedient, to tell of, to be content, to declare, to discern, to make proclamation of, to publish, to report and to witness). Suddenly, I did them and they came to pass.

4. Because I knew that you were **obstinate** (cruel, grievous, hard hearted, sorrowful, stubborn, in trouble, and unreasonably determined to have your own way), and your neck was an **iron sinew** (stubborn) and your **brow bronze** (hard headed),

5. Even from the beginning I have declared it to you. Before it came to pass I proclaimed it to you, Lest you should say, 'My idol has done them, and my carved image and my molded image have commanded them.'

6. *"You have heard; See all this. And will you not declare it? I have made you hear new things, from this time, even **hidden** (guarded, protected, maintained, preserved) things, and did you not **know** (ascertain by seeing, by recognizing, or having understanding of) them.*

7. *They are created now and not from the beginning; And before this day you have not heard them, Lest you should say, 'Of course I knew them.'*

8. *Surely you did not hear, Surely you did not know; Surely from long ago your ear was not **opened** (ungirded or unstopped), For I knew that you would deal very **treacherously** (being unfaithful, offending, and transgressing), And were called a **transgressor** (a rebel, quarreled, offended, revolted, apostatize: forsake, abandon your belief and allegiance, go beyond limits or boundaries to commit offense by violation of a law, principle, or duty) from the womb.*

9. *"For my names sake I will defer my anger, And for my praise I will restrain it from you, so that I do not cut you off.*

10. *Behold I have **refined** (purged and tried) you, but not as **silver** (but in earnest and continued inspection); I have tested you in the **furnace** (excavation) of **affliction** (depression, misery and trouble).*

11. *For My own sake, for My own sake, I will do it; For how should my name be profaned? And I will not give My glory to another.*

17. *Thus says the Lord, your Redeemer, The Holy One of Israel: "I am the Lord your God, who **teaches** (instructs, skillfully teaches) you to **profit** (set forward, to do good), Who **leads** (string a bow by treading on it, to bend, to go over, to guide, to thresh and tread down, to walk with) you by the way you should go.*

> *18. Oh that you had heeded my commandments!*
> *Then your peace would have been like a **river**
> **(flood of prosperity)**, And your **righteousness**
> **(virtue, prosperity, justice)** like the waves of the
> sea.*

The word ***"**mouth**"** found in Isaiah 48; 3 is defined in the original Hebrew as: *by means of blowing, a small wind, a spoken word, a command and an appointment.* After studying and coming to understand this interpretation of **"mouth"**, I continued to pray, and this was the answer I received.....

"The Butterfly Effect in Word"

The Butterfly Effect is used or referred to as the "Chaos Theory." It is a scientific theory that as a butterfly flitters and flutters it's wings, causing the movement of air, that movement of air, or a small wind if you will, sends out a cause and effect that may be a contributing factor to the storms in nature that lie ahead in the nearby future. Therefore, we must see that every word that proceeds from our lips, through the winds of our breath, has a cause and effect against, or for another. Our words are passed over our lips with our breath. Our breath is but, a small wind, yet still has an enormous effect on the hearts and spirits of others. The small breath that passes from our lips in the form of words, will work its effects throughout the winds until it has reached full circle, returning to us with its either damaging or building effects that it will have on the lives of others, and ultimately, the effect it will bring back to us in our own lives.

The winds of our breathed words may have a rippling effect in the lives, minds and voices of others, that may turn to a sound of thunder, bringing a devastating storm that will strike both, the lives of others, as well as our own lives, bringing about widely varied consequences ranging

An Emotional Abortion, or Emotionally Aborted?

from calamitous, dismal, or grim squalls, to gales of exhilarating, invigorating, or embracing circumstances.

Our words do change the atmosphere in us, and around us. Depending on our words, they may be tiny cultivating, enlightened changes of the atmosphere, to monstrous, ugly changes in the atmosphere that may ultimately change the path or the future of our children. Like the "Butterfly Effect," your words and your actions will affect the futures of the unborn child that grows within you.

Our words may not power or directly create the storm, but they do influence what will become your child's future. These small breaths, or winds that are formed into words, may be preventing or accelerating the storms of your child's future. Your words are the beginning and the cause of changing conditions in your child's heart and life even before it is born.

Your words will bring about changes in the initial condition of your child's heart, and your child, once born, will begin to act upon those words, bringing about a change of events or alterations that will lead to the storms of their lives. They will act upon your words in grief, pain, inadequacy, rejection, abandonment, and rebellion, or joy, exhilaration, happiness, or delight, depending on the words spoken to them, and about them. They will begin to stir the small winds of your wordy breaths, changing those wordy breaths into magnificent storms in their own lives. Will the storms of their lives be beautiful storms of love and grace, or will they be horrific storms of disgrace and evil? What words will you, or have you spoken over your child? It's not too late, no, it's never too late. God understands that we have acted out of our own wounds, pain, grief and misery. He wants to change that in you right now, if only you will let Him. I realize now, that the words I spoke over my daughter, Jeni-lee, from the moment of her conception was the very reason that she had been born with the spirit of rejection, abandonment, and rebellion. Jeni-lee, today still battles with her own demons. I believe with all my heart that her complete healing is accessible through the same

213

love, mercy, grace and understanding that the Lord has given me. Above all else, the immeasurable love for Jenilee that flows from the heart of Jesus Christ awaits her.

What kind of words have you spoken over your pregnancy(ies), or your child(ren)? If you find that you have perhaps at times, spoken unloving words (seriously or in jest), or tones of discouragement to, or about your child (ren), then now is the time to find your own root cause for the wounding words that you have sent forth to wound others. Perhaps the wounding words were spoken by the father, the grandparents, another relative, or even a friend. Perhaps you have never spoken those words over your child, or never even had a child. Perhaps you are the child that these words, or rejections have been spoken over. If so, you need to forgive them, as well as yourself. Forgiveness is the key to deliverance from our own torment and the beginning of our healing.

Unforgiveness is a self-imposed and unjust servitude to the imprisonment of grief, anger, rejection, fear, and so much more. If you feel that you are unable to forgive yourself, the father, the mother, the doctors, the nurses, or anyone else that was involved with your abortion, whether it be a physical or an emotional abortion, it will become a bondage to a life of continual loss and crippling grief.

Bondage will keep you from fully and unconditionally, loving yourself, or anyone else in your life. It is crucial to your healing that you are able to repent, confess, and forgive. After all, Jesus told us that if we do not forgive, neither, are our sins forgiven us. Matthew 6: 14, 15 says,

"For if you forgive men their trespasses, your heavenly Father will Also forgive you. "But if you do not forgive men their trespasses, Neither will your Father forgive your trespasses.

Since my abortion, all these years later, I am writing this book in the hope of educating other men and women, who have had abortions, or pregnancies that were not wanted, to let them know, they are not alone. Abortions can be a difficult thing to deal with. A very big part of me was afraid to heal, or change. I was afraid that if I gave up the grief, guilt, anger, depression, and fear, I would lose my identity. You see, I had been so wrapped up in Judith, the job , the kids, and all the drama of my life in general, I wouldn't know who I was anymore if I were to be healed and made whole again.

It's not hard to readily visualize the devastation (ruin, havoc, trauma, suffering, pain, misery) that abortion has brought into my life over the years, after reading my story.

What about you? How has abortion affected your life? I won't go on to mention the devastating effects of the emotional abortion that has fallen upon all three of my children's lives. The one thing I have to remember is that there is love, forgiveness, healing and the hope of a future, waiting for me and my children, and I pray for you too, if you will just allow it to happen.

I will no longer be a victim, but a victor! Which will you be?

If you feel that you are suffering from P.A.S., because of a choice you made, then let's begin your healing now. Please, allow me to say this prayer in agreement with you now.....

Father God, I ask You to forgive me for this calamitous sin of murder against my own flesh and blood while in my womb, and for shedding the blood of the innocent life of my unborn child. I selfishly discarded your gift of life as an inconvenience in my time of struggle. I have continued to live in the justification of my actions, and pushed forward to forget my sins against You, Oh Lord, the Creator of Life. As I have remained silent in my sin, my body, my soul and my spirit have been devastated by grief, shame, guilt, anger and condemnation. I confess my sin of murdering the innocent, and of walking in pride, instead of faith. I thank You, Jesus for having borne my griefs and carrying my sorrows. I am thankful that You, Jesus were pierced for my transgressions, crushed for my iniquities and that You made Yourself a guilt offering for my life, a punishment that is due me. I go now, to the foot of the cross where I lay down all my grief's, shame, guilt, and condemnation and I give them to you right now, Lord Jesus. Father, I ask that you restore my broken heart, and heal my shattered life, as I forgive myself and I forgive all those who took part in my sin of murdering my child in Jesus mighty name…..

I trust Lord, that my child(ren), _____ is/are now residing in Your capable hands. And now, _____, I ask for your forgiveness for taking your life instead of protecting and nurturing you into this training ground of life. I love you and I miss you, _____. I can't wait to hold you in my arms, one day soon. In a little while, we will meet again when I join you in His Kingdom, and I promise to love and cherish your precious smile, the twinkling of your eyes, and the joyous sound of your laughter. Thank you Lord Jesus for healing my heart, restoring my life, and releasing me from the bondage of self-condemnation and the spirit of death. I ask this in the unmatched, powerful name of Jesus Christ!!

Father, I come before You in faith, believing that whatever I ask in Jesus name, You will grant me. I thank You for Your revelation of the "Butterfly Effect," and the understanding of the power behind our words. I repent now, and I ask You, Lord to forgive me for the small winds, forming every word that brought calamitous disaster upon my children's hearts and their lives. I pray that all those to whom I have spoken, unaware, the evil breathy winds that formed destructive words and curses over their lives will forgive me. Teach me Lord, to love as You love, and to learn how to breathe the winds that create words of love, compassion and salvation. I recant and disavow every word spoken in my ignorance and selfishness in Jesus Mighty Name. I ask for healing of the wounded emotions I have set into action upon the hearts of my children and others, in my own selfish rebellion against You, Lord. I pray Father, that You will put a new heart in Your wounded children, and heal them with Your great compassion and love for them.

In Jesus, Precious and Holy Name
Amen

It is my prayer that you will find solace and peace in your journey of healing. You will never forget your abortion or your child. Remember, as you cry, the salt in your tears is the God given healing agent that will dry out and heal your emotional wounds. Don't be afraid or ashamed to cry, allowing all your grief and pain to escape, through your healing tears. If you need someone to talk to, be sure to look up your local pregnancy clinic and contact a grief counselor, or you can always find help through the High Desert Pregnancy Clinic by visiting their website at:

www.highdesertpregnancyclinic.org

Or you may call:

(760) 369-8512

For 24 hour emergency crisis counseling, call:

800 712 HELP (4357)

Be sure to look for

"An Emotional Healing Workbook"

By Judith Birdsong

Coming Soon!

I may be contacted at

houseofbirdsong@yahoo.com

I look forward to hearing from you!

www.ingramcontent.com/pod-product-compliance
Lightning Source LLC
Chambersburg PA
CBHW070803280326
41934CB00012B/3034